BUILDING STANDARD-BASED NURSING INFORMATION SYSTEMS

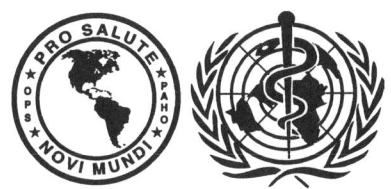

PAN AMERICAN HEALTH ORGANIZATION

Pan American Sanitary Bureau, Regional Office of the

WORLD HEALTH ORGANIZATION

DIVISION OF HEALTH SYSTEMS AND SERVICES DEVELOPMENT

ESSENTIAL DRUGS AND TECHNOLOGY PROGRAM
ORGANIZATION AND MANAGEMENT OF HEALTH SYSTEMS AND SERVICES PROGRAM
HUMAN RESOURCES DEVELOPMENT PROGRAM

PAHO Library Cataloguing in Publication Data

Pan American Health Organization.
  Building Standard-Based Nursing Information Systems
  Washington, D.C. : PAHO, © 2001. 141 p.

ISBN 92 75 12364 0

I. Title. II. Marín, Heimar F. III. Rodrígues, Roberto J.
IV. Delaney, Connie

1. INFORMATION SYSTEMS.
2. NURSING.
3. NURSING PRACTICE CLASSIFICATIONS.
4. QUALITY OF HEALTHCARE.
5. MANUALS.

NLM W26.55.I4.P187 2001

ISBN 92 75 12364 0

Cover design: Matilde Cresswell

Editors

Heimar F. Marin
Universidade Federal de São Paulo, Escola de Enfermagem, Brazil

Roberto J. Rodrigues
Health Services Information Technology (HSP/HSE), PAHO/WHO, USA

Connie Delaney
University of Iowa, College of Nursing, USA

Gunnar H. Nielsen
Danish Institute for Health and Nursing Research, Denmark
(WHO Collaborating Center for Nursing and Midwifery)

Jean Yan
Caribbean Program Coordination Office, PAHO/WHO, Barbados

Collaborators

Suzanne Bakken
Columbia University, USA

Sonia Maria Oliveira de Barros
Universidade Federal de São Paulo, Escola de Enfermagem, Brazil

Lorena Camus Bustos
Pontificia Universidad Católica, Chile

Carol Bickford
American Nurses Association, USA

Gloria H. Camargo
Fundación Santa Fé, División de Educación, Colombia

Carolina Carujo
Asociación Uruguaya de Enfermería Informática, Uruguay

Barbara Van de Castle
Johns Hopkins University, School of Nursing, USA
(PAHO/WHO Collaborating Center for Information Systems in Nursing Care)

Belkis Marcia Feliú Escalona
División de Enfermería, Ministerio de Salud Publica, Cuba

Phyllis Giovannetti
University of Alberta, Canada

Nicholas Hardiker
University of Manchester, Department of Computer Science, UK

Evelyn J.S. Hovenga
Central Queensland University,
Faculty of Informatics and Communication, Australia

Sandra Land
Organization and Management of Health Systems and Services (HSP/HSO),
PAHO/WHO, USA

Maria Lucia Lebrão
Faculdade de Saúde Pública da Universidade de São Paulo, Brazil

Carlos Hugo Leonzio
Universidade Favaloro, Argentina

Maricel Manfredi
Human Resources Development (HSP/HSR), PAHO/WHO, USA

Kathleen McCormick
SRA International Inc., USA

Randi Mortensen
The Danish Institute for Health and Nursing Research, Denmark
(WHO Collaborating Center for Nursing and Midwifery)

Susana Pepper
Departamento de Normas y Regulación, Ministerio de Salud, Chile

Virginia Saba
Georgetown University, School of Nursing, USA

Contents

Foreword

Note from the Editors

Foreword

The field of health informatics is taking center stage in the 21st century. As the information age evolves into the knowledge age, the enabling technologies will give us access to the data, information, and knowledge we need, whatever our discipline or field. Within nursing and across the healthcare team, we will look to these enablers to strengthen our ability to act knowledgeably on behalf of — and in concert with — the patient. Although informatics has already changed the way we practice our professions, we will continue our journey of transformation daily.

This journey is not local or national; it is regional and certainly global. As we work toward "better health for all," we must address similar issues and solve similar problems. Working as a team will allow us to pool our knowledge and to progress toward our shared goal. The five editors of this book have joined nineteen collaborators to form a team of twenty-four, including seven from the United States and Canada, ten from Latin America and the Caribbean, four from Scandinavia, Europe, and Australia, and three from Pan American Health Organization/World Health Organization (PAHO/WHO) in Washington, DC. We are the richer for their efforts, efforts made available and accessible to us by the publication of this book.

Because the practice and process of nursing depend heavily upon accurate and timely information, the book first focuses on standards, terminologies, and nursing information systems, and describes classification systems in nursing. Because information systems consist of "people, information, procedures, hardware, and software" working together, the book offers a discussion of nursing informatics, including such key areas as user-cordial interfaces, and privacy, security, confidentiality. Because the book reflects the wisdom of its editors and collaborators, it makes note of human and behavioral factors, notably change management and the full range of educational issues, including competencies and curriculum development.

Thus, the international team addresses both standard-based information systems and the field of nursing informatics. They have produced a book that is carefully structured, well referenced, and highly readable with key concepts displayed in text boxes.

As the recently designated PAHO/WHO Collaborating Center for Information Systems in Nursing Care at the Institute for Johns Hopkins Nursing moves forward with its work, this book will stand us in good stead. We thank PAHO/WHO for bring together the team that collaborated to produce **Building Standard-Based Nursing Information Systems**. As we work with our colleagues around the globe to improve how we serve and care for our patients, our aim is to put the ill at ease by using enabling technologies. In our journey toward the transformation of our profession—and of health care itself—this concise and timely book will serve as an invaluable roadmap and guidebook.

Marion J. Ball, EdD
Kathleen Hartman Sabatier, MS, RN

The Institute for Johns Hopkins Nursing
PAHO/WHO Collaborating Center for
Information Systems in Nursing Care

Note from the Editors

To looke upon a worke of rare devise
The which a workman setteth out to view,
And not to yield it the deserved prise,
That unto such a workmanship is dew,
Doth either prove the iudgement to be naught
Or els doth shew a mind with envy fraught.

Anonymous, *To the Learned Shepeheard (1596)*
(Commendatory sonnet in praise of
Edmund Spenser's "Faerie Queene")

Building Standard-Based Nursing Information Systems is directed to practicing and student nurses, health care professionals involved in the implementation of information systems, and information technology professionals working in the health sector.

The objective of this book is to provide them with a basic source of facts related to the use and implementation of standards in nursing clinical and administrative documentation. A compelling case is made about the importance of appropriately documenting nursing care, in order to facilitate analyses of nursing activities, the provision of quality and evidence-based direct patient care, and the promotion of continuity of service. Standardized documentation is also required for communicating nursing concepts, interventions, and outcomes to other nurses and health professionals working in different settings and countries.

The document focuses on key issues of modern nursing practice and illustrates how information technology support to the implementation and use of standard-based practice can improve clinical and management nursing functions. A review of the state of the art in nursing classifications and terminologies is presented, together with practical advice on their implementation. The extensive list of references compiled by the authors provides a rich resource for additional studies. We hope that the publication will motivate further research, will contribute to the education of nurses in standard-based practice, and assist in the development of nursing information systems in Latin America and the Caribbean.

This publication is the result of a joint initiative of three technical programs (Essential Drugs and Technology, Organization and Management of Health Systems and Services, and Human Resources Development) of the Division of Health Systems and Services Development, Pan American Health Organization, the Regional Office for the Americas of the World Health Organization. The present work was achieved over the period of one year by an intense and rewarding collaborative work with a distinguished panel of international experts followed by discussions held during and after a Caribbean Nurses Association meeting held in Trinidad and Tobago. The text was also enhanced by individual contributions included during the many revisions of the original transcripts.

We are very grateful to the professionals that collaborated in this endeavor, sharing their knowledge and experiences and unselfishly contributing their valuable time in the discussions and many revisions required in the preparation of the final copy. We could not end without a special acknowledgement to Mrs. Soledad Kearns, HSP/HSE, for her secretarial assistance in the management of the many details related to travel arrangements and in the organization of two expert technical meetings, chaired by the Regional Advisor for Health Services Information Technology, held at PAHO, in Washington, D.C.

The Editors

1.   Introduction

Nurses are the largest single group of health professionals who directly influence the quality of most health services provided and their outcomes. The area of concern of nursing ranges from clinical care of individual patients to the administration of health services and the management of health problems at all levels of complexity, including public health and community care, occupational and home care, and school health (Soberón et al., 1984).

The nursing occupation depends on accurate and timely access to appropriate information to perform the great variety of professional activities involved in patient and community care. Nursing information integrates technical knowledge, quality control, and the clinical and administrative documentation of services provided. Nurses need information about available resources, science development, and patient needs for decision making. Nurses need access to information for program planning, for the operation and supervision of clinical and management interventions and to evaluate the outcomes of care.

> *Information is a central element in decision making and an essential requisite for effective provision and management of healthcare. Access to information is recognized as a critical ingredient for health services and health program planning, operation, supervision, and control and an indispensable tool for the evaluation of clinical and managerial interventions and in the conveyance of health promotion activities (WHO, 1988; Rodrigues and Israel, 1995; WHO 1998; PAHO, 1999a; WHO, 2000).*

Computers have been recognized as an important resource to support most health technical, managerial, and knowledge-based activities, especially those that depend on current information. The importance of computers to store, retrieve, and analyze information is widely recognized. The initial motivation to develop computer systems in healthcare was driven by financial and administrative issues and automated applications were predominantly designed and deployed to target the hospital sector.

Computer-based information systems have clearly demonstrated the advances that can be achieved in effectiveness and efficiency by using appropriately designed and properly established data collection and processing systems and the implementation of data standards (McCormick, 1988; WHO, 1988; McCormick 1991; Ball, 1991a; Ball, 1991b; Sosa-Iudicissa et al., 1997; PAHO, 1998; PAHO, 1999a).

In principle, an information system does not need to be computerized. However, most of today's more complex information systems can hardly be implemented without some form of computing and telecommunications support. The degree of deployment of information systems in the health sector is, however, still quite modest. Furthermore, collected data are frequently rudimentary and of low quality when compared with data and information gathered and processed in other sectors of society, as is the case with the commercial and financial sectors, banking, agriculture, industry, tourism, insurance, and meteorology.

Computer-based applications have been developed and are widely used to produce management-oriented administrative and clinical information for operational support and decision making. Furthermore, there is an obvious explosion in the quantity of published technical information – scientific knowledge doubling about every two years (Zielstorff et al., 1993) – that cannot be managed without automated support. To achieve the full benefit of automation computerized applications must be able to communicate with each other.

There is a clear trend in the direction of the computerization of health records (Electronic Medical Record, Electronic Health Record, Computer-based Health Record, Computerized Patient Record). Economic, managerial, and regulatory determinants have been driving the convergence among ambulatory, hospital clinical records, financial records, and records of other encounters within the health system. The tendency is toward the development and eventual universal use of an individual lifelong longitudinal health record accessible to every provider independent of site of care. Moreover, the structured digitized information contained in such records would enable the use of aggregated group and population information to support public health interventions and the management of the health system.

Increasingly, more people from around the world are able to connect to the Internet. The Internet is a ubiquitous telecommunications resource that allows the fast and inexpensive exchange of data, images, and voice between a variety of electronic devices, ranging from desktop to hand-held computers and wireless devices such as pagers and telephones. As a result we can expect to see better-informed healthcare providers and consumers.

E-health is an all-inclusive term capturing the use of Internet technologies now used to describe the increasing use of electronic communication and information technologies which encompass both e-commerce (business or administrative transactions) and telehealth (clinical and educational) activities. It describes the combined use of electronic communication and information technology to transmit, store, and retrieve digital data for clinical, educational, and administrative purposes both at the local site and at a distance. Nurses must keep up, be proactive, and even assume a clear role in influencing these changes.

1.1. Information Systems and Healthcare Practice

An information system is the collection and integration of various pieces of hardware and software and the human resources that meet the data collection, storage, processing, and report generation needs of an organization. Information systems are found almost everywhere in healthcare, including hospitals, clinics, community health centers, health agencies, research facilities, and educational institutions. Their configuration, power, and functions vary widely depending on how they are used and the type of work performed in the organization (McHugh, 2001; Saba and McCormick, 2001).

Health data seldom become health information – massive amounts of data are produced and recorded in the healthcare sector, but the potentially useful information that could be generated from those data is rarely fully achieved or exploited. The key factor to the deficient use of data in the generation of information is the lack of mechanisms to process data into information and make information available in a format that is easily understood by the right people at the right time.

> *When information systems do exist, major stumbling blocks confronted by systems operators relate to the quality of data sources and timely data collection and recording. Unquestionably, data capture at the point of their generation and the accuracy issues represent the most serious concerns regarding the operation of information systems.*

Given the large quantity and the diversity of information that are required in the health sector, it is common practice to have it organized into different health information systems. When information is structured in well-defined and integrated systems, it can be collected, processed, stored, retrieved, and distributed more efficiently, and individuals and organizations will be able to use it more effectively.

1.2. Information Systems and Healthcare Organizations

Information systems are necessarily inserted in a context characterized by a variety of local needs, diverse practice environments, and levels of socioeconomic organization. Geographic environment, demographic and social determinants, economy model, political system, and the natural history of human and animal diseases pertinent to each setting influence and determine different requirements and, therefore, require different technical solutions. Epidemiological changes, life style, organizational "culture", skills and performance levels of health professionals, the regulatory and legal framework, and stage of societal development are core issues that determine the health sector organizational model and healthcare processes in each country. In addition, the globalization and internationalization of healthcare also increasingly influence all above variables. They present great challenges to health information system developers (WHO, 1988; Mandil, 1991; Rodrigues et al., 1997; PAHO, 1998; PAHO, 1999a).

In line with the social and economic changes of the last decades, most societies are presently undergoing a process of rethinking and restructuring their health organizations, management, and processes of care. In general, health sector reform experiences have been centered in changes that consider a mixed public-private practice environment, new models of patient care, the redefinition of the regulatory, provision, and financing roles of different stakeholders (the State, insurance providers, healthcare providers, regulators, and users), emphasis in accountability, the implementation of new reimbursement schemes, and maximizing technological use.

> *New models of healthcare provision encourage consultation across health disciplines and the use of inter-disciplinary and multi-disciplinary teams to provide a wider range of personal and community health services. Integrated care requires greater collaboration between health providers. Information technology applications in health are recognized as the key to providing the means of achieving cooperative integration of care, enabling services to be focused around the consumer, and reducing wasteful duplication of interventions, reporting, and expenses (Rodrigues, 2000b).*

Healthcare reform has changed the objectives of delivery systems, organizational structure, management, measurement of outcomes, and financing. Health sector reform has triggered revisions of existing laws or creation of new legislation in most countries and was a driving force in the revision of national constitutions in Argentina, Brazil, Colombia, and Mexico.

The process of change has posed great challenges – it requires political consensus, a major redefinition and realignment of management and administrative functions, increased accountability of providers, the introduction of information technology, skill development, and the development of new forms of professional education and training that stress performance and technical skills. In addition, there is a generalized need for infrastructure development through the establishment of new facilities and services to satisfy the growing user demand for efficient, cost-effective, timely, and quality care (PAHO, 2000a).

The reform processes dramatically affect health workers. Changes in personnel mix and shifting roles and responsibilities have created a number of challenges to nursing practice and to educational programs. One of the most important current trends is the concept of integrated care. In its various incarnations (managed care, comprehensive group care, etc.) this model of care has been promoted as a mean of providing better service by combining primary, secondary, and tertiary health sector interventions. Multi-disciplinary care planning and service coordination are expected to lead to improved health and well-being for people with chronic health conditions or complex care needs. Currently, for many people burdened by those health problems, care is mostly delivered by a number of quite separate service providers and funded by different levels of government and private schemes. Often the result is that people receive the care they can get rather than the care they need.

Health reform affects nursing practice and education. Nurses are being asked to initiate flexible means to update knowledge and performance in order to contribute to quality of care. In Latin America a number of trends that impact nursing educational programs have been identified: population growth, urban migration, aging populations, the increased rate of chronic and degenerative health conditions, emerging new diseases, the fast pace of health institutional and economic reforms, and the changes in family structures.

There is great variability among nursing schools and curricula. Professional skills learned and opportunities for employment are dependent on the quality and level of the educational programs. Proficiency in decision making and acquisition of technical competence to face new challenges are the major areas that must be improved in the nursing education curricula (Manfredi and Souza, 1986; PAHO, 1988).

1.3. Information Systems and Health Records

Health records are archival records or diaries of diagnostic discoveries, observations made, interventions administered, and outcomes achieved. Clinical data include facts about a patient or client's overall health status and ability to perform normal bodily functions and health records reflect a person's overall physical, physiological, psychological, sociological and intellectual characteristics and performance of interest to patients and health professionals. Health records contain time and source-oriented collections of text-based (alphanumeric) information, physiological tracings (from analogue signals), and images and sounds (multimedia).

Nurses need to be prepared to use information and telecommunications technologies to provide the best possible care for clients. Presently, many healthcare organizations are planning to implement clinical information systems including applications related to advanced electronic clinical and administrative records. Concomitantly, we are witnessing the development or upgrading of the telecommunications infrastructures around the world. These changes are enabling more people, communities, and organizations to use the Internet, videoconferencing, and related emerging technologies such as video on demand, for multiple purposes including distant education and healthcare. Educating nursing personnel in the rationale and appropriate use of information systems and in computer skills is essential to take advantage of these opportunities, as we move from an industrial economy to a knowledge-based economy.

Health records serve many different functions and information needs. When they follow a formal structure they represent individual databases consisting of a collection of discrete and ordered data elements stored in a uniform manner that permits standardized data manipulation and retrieval. Diverse combinations of data are used to produce abstracted individual patient reports for inter-professional communication as well as to provide information to a variety of direct and non-direct patient care providers for clinical and administrative decision making.

The clinical record is the main vehicle of communication of patient information among the multi-professional direct care health team members and an important tool in the evaluation and measurement of the quality of health services. Not only raw data, such as results of laboratory tests or the presence or absence of a clinical finding, but a series of interpretations, such as differential diagnoses, reasons for visit, and the physical and psychological states of a patient, need to be conveyed to a variety of providers.

Systems that process electronic versions of patient records will progressively incorporate knowledge and decision support systems to enhance clinical performance. Patients will also be interacting with the health system and its service providers differently. The adoption of computerized information systems and electronic health records will revolutionize the way everyone in the healthcare industry will work. New professional roles will be created, while others will change significantly.

New procedures and interventions will be developed. There are a variety of means by which clinically observable facts and human physical performance may be measured. Many of these tools use very sophisticated and often expensive instrumentation, which is frequently computerized. New forms of data capture will be introduced, including dynamic images of human structures and their functioning – the output of those diagnostic devices being in digitized computer-readable form. As such it should be possible to import these data directly into electronic records.

A by-product of the rigorous collection and recording of health status and nursing activity data into an electronic health record at the point of care would be the capacity to perform retrospective analyses of these data to determine the effectiveness and efficiency of medical and nursing activity in real-world settings (Roos et al., 1992). Such studies complement the use of controlled clinical trials and are related to the priorities of a practice focused on the patient and outcomes. These studies support the aims of the evidence-based best practice movement.

Evidence-based best practice may be defined as a practitioner's ability to process critical evidence and to choose interventions that are expected to achieve an optimum outcome at least risk and cost. It requires every person working in the health industry to identify the best available evidence and use this evidence as the basis for all decisions (Rodrigues, 2000c; Rodrigues, 2000d).

The corollary of deriving evidence is the production of research-based clinical guidelines to enhance nursing practice. Clinical guidelines are vital to reducing the variability in clinical nursing practice and avoiding the potentially harmful practices. The programming of computer-based decision assistance and risk-alert applications, expected to be incorporated in future practice-support information systems, is dependent on the production of research-based clinical guidelines. While such applications are presently in their infancy, their potential to improve health outcomes and prevent adverse incidents is enormous.

2. Information and Nursing Practice

The practice scope of nursing is broad, ranging from the clinical care of individual patients to the administration of health services and the management of health problems at all levels of complexity, including public health and community care, occupational and home care, and school health (PAHO, 2000b). Traditionally, most nursing activities focus on checking medical orders and procedures; however, nursing is evolving from a dependent to an independent practice.

Nursing is a profession heavily dependent on accurate and timely information. Nurses must have access to appropriate information to perform the great variety of interventions involved in nursing care. Administrative, legal, and controlling requirements; the growth of biomedical knowledge, health technologies, and therapeutic modalities; and the explosion of nursing knowledge pose increasingly complex problems. These predicaments require that nurses must integrate technical competence, quality control, and individualized patient care, and systematically improve the documentation of the whole care process. Nurses need information about available resources, science development, and patient needs – particularly, it is impossible to provide individualized care without first determining and categorizing the patient's current health status and its expected evolution. (Collier et al., 1996).

The health information required by nurses originates from a wide range of data and data sources. Health information is highly varied in nature and encompasses demographic data; information on social, cultural, economic, and environmental determinants of health; consumer preferences and lifestyle; profile of morbidity and disease-specific mortality; findings and results from clinical practice and biomedical and epidemiological research; statistics on the activities of healthcare services; actions of health personnel; coverage of health programs; and individual patient health data sources including patient records and files, with all their complex and diverse contents (e.g., diagnostic laboratory numerical and text results, electrocardiograms, images, etc.)

2.1.   Problems of Clinical and Administrative Records

Nurses face several constraints in the documentation and recovery of information. Although nurses spend from eight to thirty percent of their time in data-related tasks (Carpenito, 1997), there is a significant shortfall in the quality, and sometimes in the quantity, of nursing activities recorded in the clinical and administrative documentation. Even when data are effectively captured, few are processed into meaningful information (Rodrigues and Israel, 1995; Rodrigues et al., 1995; PAHO, 1998; Herrero et. al., 1998; WHO, 2000).

> *The documentation of nursing interventions is one of the weakest components of the nursing care process. Underlying causes for this problem are related to the insufficient number of providers relative to the patient demands, lack of time to record the details of care provided, and the absence of structured forms for data collection and of a comprehensive system for data processing and retrieval.*

Documentation of clinical and administrative data is varied and complex in nature. With the expansion of health data and information in clinical and administrative practice, nursing documentation increases in volume and level of detail without concomitant improvement in the quality of informational content. Accurate recording is resource and time intensive. This situation is not expected to improve. Today's healthcare environment increasingly demands the development of professional and efficient documentation systems for concurrent use by a variety of health professionals.

Ideally, data should be collected at the point of care, otherwise it will take more time and resources to find, record, retrieve, and analyze clinical and administrative data. Registering data some time after care is provided, for example at the end of a shift, may also compromise the quality of data and information may be lost or forgotten.

Significant clinical and administrative data and information frequently do not find their way into the individual health record. Consequently, important patient and intervention data are missing. Many patient records do not include evidence of the contribution of nursing care to the outcome of treatment. Nursing practice should be underpinned by evidence-based nursing research. However, to conduct research, there is a need for nursing documentation to support data retrieval and analysis.

It is difficult, if not impossible, to clarify and quantify nursing contribution to the health of individuals and the population. Data that are not properly documented obviously cannot be used to demonstrate nursing performance, the cost of nursing care, or the evidence of best practice.

2.2. Nursing Documentation in Latin America and the Caribbean

In developing countries, low priority is given to medical records because incentives such as legal, reimbursement, accreditation, and other requirements that are based on an appropriately completed health record do not exist or are not enforced.

Less-qualified nursing staff, such as nurse assistants and aides, that usually represent the bulk of health professionals in developing countries, receive only a basic level of training. This level of training does not enable them to deliver and document nursing care appropriately and to follow the Nursing Process – a systematic problem-oriented decision making process of organizing and delivering nursing care. Consequently, nursing care is fragmented, procedure-focused, and difficult or impossible to analyze in terms of quality and cost-benefit.

Agreement regarding the structure of the nursing documentation, vocabularies, and the quality of recorded data is recognized as a major problem in Latin America and the Caribbean (Angerami and Carvalho, 1987; Anselmi et al., 1988; Gir et al., 1990; Dias, 1990; Simões, 1992; Yoshioca et al., 1993). The issues are magnified by a number of factors (Manfredi, 1993; PAHO, 1999b) including:

- High demand for nursing care;

- Insufficient number of registered nurses;

- Wide disparity in means, levels, and quality of professional education and performance;

- Most nursing care delivered by nursing assistants or aides;

- Specific requirements for documentation of care according to each agency, institution, level of professional education, tradition, routines, and legal environment rather than standardized documentation;

- Lack of recognition of nursing documentation as an important aspect to explain and characterize nursing contribution to the healthcare;

- Absence of documentation in standard format precludes extraction for analysis;

- Different classification systems originating from other countries that frequently are not pertinent to the local users and pattern of care;

- Lack of validation and evaluation of classification systems;

- Lack of standard data and standard sets of nursing care terms or terminologies to support the implementation of the Nursing Process;

- Absence of benchmarking methodologies and tools for quality and cost-effectiveness of nursing care;

- Lack of experience in managing complex organizations, a changing environment and multi-professional teams;

- Lack of knowledge and skills relative to information technology and low motivation to learn about technology complicated by lack of its recognition as an essential personal asset in the evaluation of professional performance;

- Lack of integrated automated health information systems in health organizations;

- Nursing documentation frequently not included as a component of automated health information systems.

Nurses must recognize the importance of data and information that document contribution to patient care and must continue to focus on refining and standardizing documentation to demonstrate their role in assisting the patient toward recovery, stabilization of health, or a peaceful death (Iyer and Camp, 1999). Currently, topics that address those issues are being introduced in the curriculum of nursing education programs in the Region.

3.   The Nursing Process

This section describes how the Nursing Process may be used as a vehicle for the delivery of nursing care. It also explains how elements of the nursing process may be used to provide a structural framework for the nursing record – a framework that presents a clear account of the care given to individual patients/clients.

The American Nurses Association (ANA, 1998a) defines nursing as the diagnosis and treatment of human responses to actual or potential health problems. It is also assumed that nursing care is individualized to meet a particular patient's unique needs and situation. The Nursing Process is a rational evidence-based methodology for the provision of nursing care. The Nursing Process adds accountability to the professional practice.

> *To support nursing care practice, the Nursing Process methodology has been used as a useful instrument valid across different countries and healthcare delivery models. The Nursing Process is recognized as a universal methodology to organize and perform nursing care. It is a framework within which nurses can organize information about patient problems and design interventions to meet their needs.*

3.1.   Explaining the Nursing Process

Nursing is a complex and challenging discipline mostly because nurses deal with more than just diseases and technology and deal with the full range of human responses to actual or potential health problems (Friedlander, 1981; Collier et al., 1996; Villalobos, 1999). Several themes cut across all areas of nursing practice and reflect nursing responsibilities for every type of patients. These themes provide an additional dimension for attention and inclusion. In this context, it is obligatory to consider that a more scientific and complex approach to the nursing care process is required. The role of information technology is vital. Nursing knowledge feeds nursing information systems and vice versa. The technological advances have been pushing nurses to evaluate our knowledge base and have given the profession a multiplicity of new resources that can be exploited in delivering better patient care.

The Nursing Process is an assertive, problem-solving approach to the identification and treatment of client problems and an important tool for nursing education. This process requires the early development of a series of abilities and capacities and an appropriate knowledge base in students and practitioners (Zaragoza, 1999). The Nursing Process encompasses all significant decision making and actions by nurses in the provision of care to all clients, and forms the foundation for clinical decision making. It focuses on the activities and interventions of the healthcare provider, services performed, or the process of nursing care. Nurses assess, diagnose, intervene, and evaluate (Lang and Brooten, 1999).

The five-step Nursing Process is the foundation of clinical decision making and encompasses all significant steps taken by nurses in providing care (Doenges et al., 1995; ANA, 1998a):

(a) Nursing Assessment - a systematic and ongoing collection of data relating to the patient; pertinent data are collected using appropriate assessment techniques; relevant data are documented in a retrievable form. Data may include the following dimensions: physical, psychological, social, cultural, spiritual, cognitive, functional abilities, developmental, economic, and lifestyle.

(b) Problem Identification or Diagnosis - consists of the analysis of the collected assessment data to identify the patient's problems/diagnoses, needs, and resources. Diagnoses are documented in a manner that facilitates the determination of expected outcomes and plan of care. Identified accepted outcomes that are individualized to the patient and documented as measurable goals are included. Outcomes provide direction for continuity of care.

(c) Planning - developing a plan of care that prescribes interventions to attain expected outcomes; i.e. linkages are established among diagnoses, interventions, and outcomes. The plan is individualized to the patient and priorities for care reflecting current practice are established.

(d) Implementation - identified interventions are carried out, the plan of care is put into action, and the interventions are documented in a timely manner. Activities may include any or all of these actions: intervening, delegating, and coordinating.

(e) Evaluation - the accuracy of diagnoses and effectiveness of the interventions are evaluated in relationship to the patient's progress; actual outcomes are determined. The effectiveness of interventions is documented in relation to the attainment of the outcomes.

Many care centers and hospitals all over the world are striving to implement the Nursing Process in order to establish a methodology to deliver evidence-based nursing care. However, there is a common tendency to put into practice just the nursing assessment and diagnosis components, removed from the context of the Nursing Process as a whole. One must stress the planning, implementation, and evaluation phases, where nursing interventions and outcomes are selected and performed, taking into account the identified nursing diagnoses. Nurse interventions correlated with patient's outcomes are one of the most important sources of data for the analysis of the effectiveness of treatments and benefits of nursing care and for the measurement of the nursing contribution to the health of the population.

In the U.S., the five steps of the Nursing Process have been expanded to six and include an optional step – *Outcome Identification* (ANA, 1998a) placed between the *Planning* and the *Implementation* steps:

(f) ***Outcome Identification*** - expected outcomes are individualized to the patient and are derived from the diagnoses. They include a time estimate for attainment, are used to provide direction for continuity of care, and are documented as measurable goals to be reached and evaluated.

3.2. Standard Terminologies

The traditional method of describing nursing care, i.e., providing the data to populate the nursing record, takes the form of hand-written notes, also known as unstructured text. There are many advantages to this approach. Unstructured text is very flexible. It is, for instance, possible to describe the same concepts in many different ways, e.g. "*Severe Pain*" or "*Agony*". It is also possible to describe the same concepts at various levels of detail: from a very high-level, e.g. "*Mr. Garcia has suffered a severe and acute abdominal pain in the right lower quadrant since 23:00h last night*" to a general statement, e.g. "*Patient states that he has pain in his abdomen*". A further benefit to this approach is that it requires no change in the way we generally think about patient information. However, the problems with unstructured text are determined to a large extent by these same properties of flexibility and expressiveness. The ability to describe identical concepts in different ways impairs communication of exact meanings, makes comparisons of nursing care difficult, and hinders analysis of nursing data.

> *The problems related to the use of unstructured text are magnified by the use of computers and have fuelled the development of a number of structured terminologies, i.e., predefined and agreed-upon sets of terms that describe in a consistent way important nursing concepts for nursing diagnoses, nursing interventions, and so forth. The major purpose of an agreed-upon structured terminology is to demonstrate the value of nursing and its contribution to health care. A standard terminology allows itself to be coded, stored, and retrieved in a usable format.*

Several national and international nursing organizations have identified a need for standardized terminologies to describe, compare, and communicate nursing care activities across settings, population groups, and countries (Gassert, 1998). They further determined that the nursing caregivers need reliable data to formulate health policy and to develop standards for computer-based information systems. The International Council of Nurses (ICN) agreed that the need for a common language for nursing was urgent if nursing wanted to be an integral part of the computer-based information systems being developed for the healthcare delivery system in the 21st century.

3.3. Documenting the Nursing Process

Assuming that the Nursing Process is indeed an appropriate framework for nursing practice, the internal structuring of the nursing documentation should be based on that model. The characteristics of the nursing professional activities, the framework for nursing practice, and the sequential phasing of the Nursing Process emphasize that one of the main professional functions of nurses is the monitoring and evaluation of the patient's responses to nursing interventions. The clinical and administrative documentation must clearly communicate a nurse's judgment and evaluation of the patient's status. The ability of the nursing professional to make a difference in patient outcomes must be demonstrated in practice and reflected in charting (Iyer and Camp, 1999).

> *Documentation is the evidence that the nurse's legal and ethical responsibilities to the patient were met and that the patient received care of acknowledged quality. Florence Nightingale (1820-1910), a British nurse who in 1854 organized and directed a unit of field nurses during the Crimean War, is considered the founder of modern nursing. She was the first nurse to emphasize how important it is to document nursing care. Since then, nurses have viewed documentation as a vital part of professional practice and recognized it as a way to evaluate nursing care.*

The increasingly complex healthcare needs of patients and shortened lengths of stay have highlighted the need for efficient collection of data. Ideally, structured forms should be used to facilitate data collection. The forms to collect data must reflect identified patient's needs and facilitate the elaboration of accurate nursing diagnoses and priority setting to guide the selection of interventions.

Documentation forms must be easy to use, friendly, driven by clinical characteristics, and useful to the all-important requirement of allocating nursing time effectively. Priority should be given to the design of forms and databases for the most frequently seen problems in the general population expected to use the health service. Specific data related to less usual health problems and clinical specialties will be added as required in order to build a comprehensive record. Some areas such as public health, community health, occupational health, home care, and school health will require the creation of forms that require very specific data elements appropriate to each setting.

The initial encounter with the patient should focus on the following four priorities for assessment: *Problems*, *Patient's Risk for Injury* (e.g., falls, ulcers, and violence), *Potential for Self-care Following Discharge* and *Patient and Family Education Needs* (Iyer and Camp, 1999).

In the *first phase* of the Nursing Process, the assessment must include data and information to support the identification of the patient's needs. All subsequent phases of the Nursing Process depend on the quality of the initial assessment and respective documentation. Several sources in the extensive literature on nursing documentation discuss in detail the requirements of documentation for the assessment phases. A summary of the most significant issues that must be considered follows:

- Describe the findings in such way that all providers can easily understand;

- Avoid interpretation describing what is seen, heard, and felt according to the patient's description and, as much as feasible, using patient's own words;

- Document symptoms that the patient denies and the negative findings as well as positive symptoms and findings; negative findings can, frequently, assist in reaching the proper diagnoses;

- If the patient cannot answer questions or provide information in the assessment interview, document the reasons;

- Make sure that patient allergies are documented in an explicit and easily seen way for all providers.

The *second phase* of the Nursing Process involves problem identification or diagnosis, needs, and expected required human and material resources. Signs, symptoms, and associated factors can provide evidence of the diagnosis or diagnoses. They are documented in order to spell out and justify the clinical judgment that was made by the responsible nurse. Frequently, a variety of psychosocial, cultural, economic, cognitive, developmental, and lifestyle-related factors can reflect different physiologic responses and modify the form and resources that must be mobilized to deal with the identified health problem. In addition, the documentation of the nursing diagnosis should also reflect the desired outcomes. Knowing the patient needs, outcomes can be established in order to provide mechanisms for evaluating the patient's progress and the effectiveness of the interventions delivered to address the identified diagnoses.

The *third* and *fourth phases* of the Nursing Process are, respectively, the planning and the implementation of required interventions. Nursing interventions have to be specific to the identified diagnosis. The interventions are meant to direct the care provided by the nursing staff and should include their frequency. The use of action verbs is mandatory in describing the proposed interventions in order to guide the execution of the correct intervention and avoid errors. In addition, all interventions should be dated and signed by the nurse who prescribed them. Interventions are individualized according to the patient needs. However, they should be also realistic for the patient and nurse, considering the length of stay, the resources available, and the expected outcomes (Iyer and Camp, 1999). The documentation of the implemented interventions is done in the nursing progress notes of the patient record, whether in manual or electronic format. These observations are related to the identified diagnosis and the performed related interventions and should reflect the response or the status of the patient related to the specific care.

Finally, in the *fifth phase*, the evaluation of the patient's status is conducted. This is a most important ongoing part of the Nursing Process. Clearly defined outcomes direct how and when to evaluate the achievement of expected outcomes. They provide a framework for the documentation of the achievement of the expected outcomes. Outcomes are increasingly being used as a tool to evaluate the performance of the nursing staff and serve as a basis for comparison of patient care with other healthcare organizations, departments, clinics, or agencies.

> *Where possible, nurses are advised to develop paper-based documentation systems that permit an easy transfer to computerized systems. The Nursing Process methodology provides a good foundation for the development of standardized forms. Forms must use a standardized terminology of defined terms. Terminologies must be selected considering user acceptance and their ability to support quality detailed documentation of care appropriate for each area of application.*

As far as possible the terms used to describe and document nursing practice should reflect the language commonly used by all nurses to ensure system adoption and acceptance. This then becomes the basis for an information system user interface, i.e., data readable via a computer, to be mapped to a standard reference terminology within the system. Such mapping permits variations between user interfaces regarding the terms used without compromising the ability to compare or aggregate data retrieved from any number of other systems.

In nursing, major efforts have been made to document and classify the structures and processes of care and to link those processes to resulting outcomes. The use of standardized terminologies facilitates communication between nurses and other health professionals, makes it easier to compare nursing practice within a particular setting and across diverse settings, and provides the foundation for data aggregation, analysis, and measurement of outcomes (Saba, 1999). The next chapter will describe in more detail terminologies and the structures that underpin them. Moreover, it identifies structures that make terminologies useful.

3.4. Quality Assurance

Quality assurance is a continuous and lifelong professional mandate and the essential component of a quality assurance model. It involves deciding on standards and guidelines that represent quality care, including data on these quality measures in patient records; measuring care given and received; and taking action to assure quality care.

Quality assurance programs, in general, examine the care given to groups of patients and individuals. When dealing with patient groups, similar patients are selected based on a common socioeconomic characteristics, health problem, medical diagnosis, nursing diagnosis or intervention, or medical or surgical procedure. Examples of way to group patients include degree of wellness, pain, incontinence, lack of knowledge, child abuse, etc. Adequate documentation and classification are essential for this work.

> *Outcomes such as mortality and morbidity are well-understood measures but may not be particularly informative for understanding the effects of nursing interventions. Outcome measures more sensitive to the effects of nursing actions are needed, such as functional, physiological, and psychological status; stress level; satisfaction with care received; symptom control; home functions; caregiver burden; goal attainment; quality of life; utilization of service; safety; and cost of care.*

More recently, researchers working with large national data sets have been attempting to identify quality-nursing indicators that can be associated with patients' outcomes (ANA, 1997; Lang and Brooten, 1999).

4. Standards, Terminologies, and Nursing Information Systems

This chapter focuses on *standards* and *structured terminologies* and how they might be used to document the Nursing Process as well as populate nursing minimum data sets, i.e., core sets of essential data that have been grouped together to serve a specific purpose or set of purposes.

> *A standard is a set of rules, guidelines, or desired characteristics for physical objects, materials, activities, behaviors, performance, quality, or their results, which are consolidated in a technical document and aimed at the achievement of an optimum degree of order in the functioning of any equipment, procedure, system, or organization. Standards are evolutionary in nature. They are established by consensus, and approved by a peer-recognized professional or technical body of experts, or by a regulatory or governmental agency. It is expected that standards will be used universally for the specific area where they apply. For a given context, information system standards address issues of order and compatibility in the design, development, implementation, and operation of information systems and information technology.*

When talking about standards in nursing, one must, distinguish between *standards of nursing practice,* aimed toward the achievement of quality and excellence in professional practice, and *standards needed to build quality information systems for the support of nursing practice.*

4.1. Practice Standards and Information Systems Standards

A *standard for clinical nursing practice* can be described as a document established by consensus among nurses and approved by a recognized body, e.g., a healthcare authority, setting down rules or guidelines aimed at the achievements of the optimum degree of excellence in the area of clinical nursing practice. Nursing practice standards describe the professional responsibilities of all nurses for every practice setting (ANA, 1998). Standards of nursing practice are authoritative statements that describe the level of care and desired common performance for the profession and by which the quality of nursing practice can be assessed. Nursing standards also describe the process of providing care through the use of the Nursing Process (standards of care) and the accomplishment of professional activities (standards of performance).

Standards needed to build information systems for the support of nursing practice are concerned with nursing concepts[1] and data. Standards of relevance to nursing information systems can be identified as necessary in the design and development of the different components of information systems: hardware; generic software; and application software, including the logical model used in the development of the application and the user interface levels. The discussion that follows will focus on the logical level description of nursing information systems and corresponding standards.

4.2. Standards in Nursing Information: Concepts and Data

Among the *information system standards* that are pertinent to the logical level of systems design, a distinction must be made between *standards related to concepts* and *standards related to data*. This important distinction is reflected in the design of nursing terminologies, in particular the distinction between a *combinatorial terminology* (that addresses concepts) and an *enumerative terminology* (that addresses data-related issues).

Two examples illustrate how this difference in perspective determines how terminologies are developed and used:

---

[1] Here it should be noted that *concepts* (a unit of thought) are expressed by *terms* (a unit of language) and that *systems of concepts* are expressed by terminologies. The expression "*standards for a system of concepts*" is therefore synonymous to the expression "*standards for terminologies*".

- In *combinatorial terminologies* a number of simple (atomic) concepts combine into complex (molecular) concepts. As examples, the two atomic concepts "*sleep*" and "*disturbed*" may combine into the complex concept "*disturbed sleep*" and the two simple concepts "*acute*" and "*pain*" may similarly come together to become the complex concept "*acute pain*". Combinatorial classification systems have helped to disseminate the notion of concepts and their combinations, and promoted the implementation of concept standards. They have been used to describe the structural features of nursing concepts systems and terminologies in nursing classification systems.

- *Enumerative terminologies*, on the other hand, assume that concepts are pre-combined into complex concepts. The concepts "*disturbed sleep*" and "*acute pain*" are examples of such data items. Traditional nursing concept systems or terminologies use enumerative data models typically represented by lists of relevant data items.

Building a standard-based nursing information systems means building nursing information systems that use *nursing concept* standards and *nursing data* standards. Developing nursing information systems in the age of modern information technology also implies building systems that take into account standards concerned with structural aspects, of a more technical nature, i.e., related to the inherent characteristics and requirements of computer-based systems as the apply to both data and terminologies.

There are many standards on different possible levels of description of nursing practice and activities but, currently, the development of nursing information systems emphasizes four areas defined by the pairs *Concept/Data* and *Structure/Content*. They are summarized in the following table:

	STRUCTURE	CONTENT
Concept Standards	Categorial Structures and Formal Terminology Models in Nursing	Nursing Concepts in Systems/Terminologies (Nursing Classification Systems)
Data Standards	Data and Information Models in Nursing	Nursing Data Sets

4.3. Structured Terminologies

4.3.1. Simple Lists

The straightforward solution to the dilemma of using unstructured text in contemporary computerized nursing information systems is to standardize a terminology. This is accomplished by agreeing in advance on all of the expressions we might want to use, and by presenting these expressions in a list (Figure 1). Describing nursing care is just a case of selecting all relevant expressions from the list and transcribing them into the nursing record or even selecting them from a pick list on a computer screen.

Figure 1. A Simple List

Acute abdominal pain
Acute pain
Pain
Severe pain
Chronic pain

Since the set of terms is predetermined, the use of such a terminology in a particular setting, locality, or region provides a common basis for describing nursing care. However, in constructing any predefined set of expressions, developers must limit the number of expressions they might include, so that the total number of expressions remains manageable, both in terms of development and in terms of effort needed to retrieve or "look up" the expressions. It soon becomes obvious that the number of expressions actually needed to describe nursing care is unmanageable. Moreover, in simple lists there are no mechanisms for aggregating or grouping terms, which results in major difficulties with the organizing, accessing, retrieving, and analyzing information. For example, there is no way to identify that the expression "*Pain*" is related to the more detailed expression "*Severe pain*" and "*Acute abdominal pain*".

4.3.2. Classifications

One solution to the problem of aggregating or grouping terms to allow the proper organization, access, and analysis of information is to organize expressions into a classification scheme (Figure 2). Classifications are terminology systems in which predefined expressions are related by hierarchical relationships. The majority of commonly reported standardized nursing terminologies take this form.

Figure 2. Classification

```
1.     Pain
1.1.   Acute pain
1.1.1. Acute abdominal pain
1.2.   Severe pain
1.2.1. Severe abdominal pain
 .
 .
 .
```

Classification schemes purport to provide a mechanism for:

- Formalizing and expanding knowledge about nursing practice;

- Helping to determine the cost of nursing services;

- Helping to target resources more effectively;

- Making explicit the role of nurses in healthcare.

Classifications have a useful role in data retrieval analysis. They facilitate further reuse of data by being able to be linked to a range of knowledge sources such as decision-support systems, therapeutic protocols, and practice guidelines. Classifications are also seen as useful for statistical evaluation through several important characteristics:

- Stability is required to allow comparative analysis over time;

- It should be possible to place any relevant expression within a category. In order to guarantee exhaustiveness, classifications may provide both common categories and catch-all categories such as "*Not otherwise specified*";

- Classifications must guarantee mutual exclusivity to avoid double counting;

- Classifications require rules to maintain consistency in their use.

These characteristics require that classifications should not include too much detail. This makes classifications particularly suitable to the recording of minimum data sets, which have been defined with more statistically-oriented tasks in mind. However, with respect to patient care there is increasing evidence to show that existing classifications are not able to represent the kind of nursing data commonly recorded in patient records in sufficient detail. They may be poorly suited to describing and documenting day-to-day nursing care – as in the case of simple lists; the number of expressions needed to describe nursing care in any detail becomes quickly unmanageable.

A number of problems, however, plague the development and implementation of classification schemes in the health sciences. Any classification of biomedical phenomena tends to be both *shallow*, and therefore the terms are confined to a somewhat coarse-grained and abstract level, and *narrow*, i.e., tuned to a single purpose or to a group of closely related purposes. In addition, the expressions in such terminologies may be quite unnatural to users, as they require the categorization of concepts in a definitive manner, while clinical expressions are often too ambiguous for such an endeavor. Also, the arrangement of expressions into hierarchies is also challenging – if the total number of expressions must be limited, then the number of expressions at any particular level must also be limited. Moreover, there are potentially many ways to classify any individual expression. For example, is *"pre-operative anxiety"* a kind of anxiety, or a kind of pre-operative problem?

Finally, both simple lists and classifications are difficult to extend. For example, if one wants to add a general modifier to all expressions in a list or classification one would need to redefine these expressions so that they include all of the values for that modifier.

4.3.3. Combinatorial Terminologies

An alternative to the use of lists and classifications is the use of combinatorial terminologies (Figure 3) where complex expressions are broken down into simpler or atomic concepts. These concepts are usually organized into a set of axes, to reflect the nature of the original source expressions.

Figure 3. Combinatorial Terminology

FOCUS	ONSET	SITE	SEVERITY
Pain	Acute	Abdomen	Severe
	Chronic	Chest	Mild

The different axes within combinatorial terminologies may be presented as simple lists or as classifications. Thus the ability to combine more elementary concepts into more complex content areas creates the potential to generate expressions with a very high degree of detail. In this way, combinatorial terminologies attempt to address some of the inherent problems of lists and classifications.

Despite their strengths, combinatorial terminologies are awkward for direct use:

- They require multiple selections from a series of different lists or classifications.

- Current computerized or manual implementations that provide a framework for reconstructing complex clinical expressions are impaired by the lack of specific rules for determining which combinations are clinically reasonable and for determining canonical (approved, authoritative) forms for concepts.

- Combinatorial terminologies can neither prevent the creation of clinically meaningless concepts nor control the great number of possible combinations of terms (combinatorial explosion).

- Complex concepts are difficult to classify, and by necessity, the hierarchical relationships between concepts must be inferred when retrieving is done. Combinatorial terminologies cannot maintain this kind of inference themselves, and they must rely on computer systems to manage this process (Button et al., 1998).

4.3.4. Formal Terminologies

Another alternative is the use of advanced computer-based formal systems. A formal terminology is built upon a terminology model, i.e., a set of high-level categories and the relationships between them. It incorporates a set of expressions, which represent atomic or single concepts. Formal terminologies use a prescriptive knowledge representation, i.e., a predetermined sequence of instructions that encode the facts that must be represented, which can be supported by software tools. Those tools are responsible for the management and manipulation of the terminology, including the recognition of redundancy, equivalence, and automatic classification.

While formal terminologies offer great sophistication, power, and flexibility, there is a trade-off – formal terminologies are complex and depend on computer support. They are also difficult to develop, maintain, and implement. The low level of sophistication of many nursing information systems products and the continuing requirement for paper-based models should not be overlooked, and there is a continuing need for simpler purpose-specific terminologies for the foreseeable future.

4.4. Developing Standards

Independent groups, professional associations, academic institutions, and government agencies work with interested health providers and informatics experts toward the establishment and refinement of health information standards. Work in progress recognizes internationally standards already established and do not seek to recreate standards that have a fair degree of readiness and market acceptance. At country level, a National Standards Organization examines, evaluates, and controls the formal process for the acceptance and publication of standards.

> *Professional organizations and bodies, like the International Council of Nurses (ICN) and the World Health Organization (WHO), and technology-oriented standardization organizations, like the International Standardization Organization (ISO) and the Comité Europeen de Normalisation (CEN), are the most important source of health standards. In 1998, the International Standards Organization (ISO) established a technical committee (TC-215) to specifically deal with health informatics standards. It now has several active technical subcommittees and works closely with similar groups such as the European CEN TC251. Nurses may be represented via any number of organizations.*

A terminology of reference is the keystone in building informatics applications that will use clinical data to learn from and improve practice and nurse researchers from around the world have agreed to collaborate in the development of an all-encompassing nursing terminology model of reference. This work will eventually set up a nursing terminology for international use that will be consistent with the goals and objectives of all existing health terminology models contributing to the establishment of a unified healthcare model representation. The international nursing terminology model is expected to embody the knowledge and representation of:

- Nursing concepts (definition of *categorical structures and formal terminology model*),

- The relationships of core concepts to essential attributes or properties (*semantic relationships* that result in a classification system),

- The definition of data structures (*data model*), and

- The definition of nursing data required (*data sets*).

The intent of this comprehensive terminology is to capture the full range of nursing concepts and definitional relationships in all areas of general and specialized practice and in all regions, countries and cultures. The concepts and relationships of the model will be specific to nursing knowledge and practice but are likely to overlap to some degree with concepts and relationships used by other patient care disciplines. By providing a defining structure for nursing core concepts and their relationships to essential attributes or properties, the terminology model of reference will provide a common framework for the many nursing terminologies in use around the world and will help the building, maintenance, and mapping between different terminologies. The terminology model of reference will also provide the basis for valid comparisons of nursing practice presently expressed and recorded in distinct terminologies that reflect the colloquial usage in different countries and cultures.

Recently, a first working document for international standards related to the structural features of nursing concept systems and nursing terminologies has been published by the Comité Européen de Normalisation (CEN, 2000). A related initiative, concerned with structural aspects of nursing concept systems and terminologies, is in progress within the framework of the International Standardization Organization (ISO) in its Workgroup 3 (Concept Representation).

Many researchers and healthcare providers have argued that a variety of terminologies are needed to cover the entire breadth of nursing, and that no one terminology can possibly meet all the needs of all nurses. The existence of different structured terminologies for nursing would appear to contradict the desire for more effective communication, a standardized firm foundation for data aggregation and analysis, and the development of tools capable of providing comparisons of nursing practice.

Terminology standards are technical standards and as such they do not intrude on the professional issue of content. Through the definition of agreed terminology models, derived from existing nursing terminologies, terminology standards seek to reduce any unnecessary diversity between terminologies.

> *To address the problems arising from the proliferation of nursing terminologies, a number of organizations are collaborating in the development of standards to underpin the full range of structured nursing terminologies. These standards deal with the essential structure of terminologies.*

Related standards, intrinsic to the field of health information, are also being developed to support information systems development and information sharing among different subsystems and applications. They must be taken into account in the logical design of databases and may be specific to the particular information system, institutional environment, and model of care. Examples of such standards include: identifier standards (patient, provider, site-of-care, product and supply labeling), message format standards, content and structure standards, clinical data representations (codes), confidentiality and data security, and data quality standards (see Appendix 3.)

4.5.   Criteria for Selecting a Standardized Terminology

For a terminology to be of value it must meet the two criteria of being *usable* and *useful*.

To be *usable*, a terminology must be appropriate to the cognitive skills and training of users and the infrastructure resources and match the organizational context of its use. Computer-based terminologies that depend on software tools for their management are not applicable where the required technology is not available. Even the use of paper-based terminologies may not be possible if they are not accompanied by appropriate support to ensure adequate speed of use, accuracy, and comprehensiveness. In addition, terminologies based on a particular culture (e.g., terminologies that support a particular nursing model) may not be easily translated into other cultures.

> *Terminologies are highly dependent on their intended purpose and why and how they will be used. In reality, an individual terminology can serve many different purposes. Each particular purpose will require some degree of trade-off. For example, for the specific task of capturing day-to-day nursing care, there is an inevitable compromise to be made between level of detail and simplicity of use. For statistical evaluation the fact that the terminology used may not be appropriate for describing day-to-day care must be taken into account as it may affect how efficiently data are collected and the accuracy of conclusions drawn from data analysis.*

To be *useful*, a terminology must be in a form and contain all of the features relevant to the task or tasks in hand. These tasks might include populating standardized care plans, providing descriptions for referrals, charting exceptions to critical paths, providing appropriate aggregations for reporting incidence of nursing diagnoses, indexing bibliographic sources, etc. The terminology should be broad enough. It should cover the particular area of interest. The terminology should also be detailed enough; it should accommodate an appropriate level of detail. In order to handle minor variations in practice or local nuances, the terminology should allow for local extensions, without compromising the integrity of the terminology or diminishing its value in carrying out the task.

Any nursing terminology should of course be appropriate for the domain or for particular subspecialties of the nursing profession. The language used or generated should be readily understandable to users and it should accurately reflect current nursing practice. On a more technical note any relationships within the terminology should be consistently applied.

If comparisons are required, either a particular terminology should be agreed across the relevant setting, locality, or region, or accurate mappings should be available across the terminologies involved to an agreed target terminology. These mappings should be sufficiently sensitive and specific to meet all intended purposes. To facilitate comparison, the possibility of describing the same concept in different ways (redundancy) and of describing different concepts using the same expression (ambiguity) should be minimized. Moreover, precise context-independent definitions should form an integral part of the terminology.

4.6. Nursing Minimum Data Sets

Nursing data represent the primary level of nursing informatics. Nursing data are the basic tool used to elaborate and record the Nursing Process through the methodology of assessment, diagnoses, interventions, outcomes, documentation, and evaluation of patient care. According to Saba and McCormick (1996), nursing data are defined and coded terms are needed for the development of computer-based information systems. Nursing data, once processed, produce nursing information, and nursing information, once analyzed, interpreted, and aggregated, produces nursing knowledge.

Nursing Information means data captured, organized, and interpreted. Consequently, an information system refers to the processing of data elements that are stored in a database into information (Saba and McCormick, 1996; Saba and McCormick, 2001). The processing of information, much more complex than the processing of data, results in the development of new information (information in context), a higher-level product representing aggregated information from different sources.

In recent years a great focus of interest in the nursing profession is to determine what kind of data are essential to guarantee nursing care. The question is which data elements are required to describe nursing diagnoses, interventions, and outcomes. The discussion now is moving professionals around the world because, if there are no data that reflect nursing judgments about patient problems/needs, interventions and activities, or outcomes, there will be no archival record of what nurses do, what difference nursing care makes, or why nurses are required.

Nurses need data for clinical decision making about the allocation and management of scarce resources. Beyond economic survival, nurse administrators need accurate and reliable data to manage quality and determine the adequacy of care. The determination of client outcomes is linked to provider actions, yet is complicated by the lack of agreement on the definitions and measures of intervening contextual co-variates derived from the setting in which care is delivered (Rodrigues and Goihman, 1990; Huber and Delaney, 1998).

Outcomes can best be understood when data about both the nursing care delivered and the nursing delivery system are available. It is necessary to look at the contextual framework of care to reliably determine the effectiveness of patient outcomes. For example, the impact of unit size, staff ratios and turnover, education and experience, work intensity, and costs on patient outcomes must be determined. Capturing these data will assist in studying clinical nursing outcomes within context.

The pioneering development in the identification of core nursing data elements was led by Werley in 1988, who defined the Nursing Minimum Data Set (NMDS) as "a minimum set of items of information with uniform definitions and categories concerning the specific dimension of professional nursing, which meets the information needs of multiple data users in the healthcare system" (Werley and Lang, 1995).

> *In addition to the development of uniform definitions for the data elements, standardized classification systems continue to be developed for each data element to support the collection of uniform and accurate data. However, it is necessary to emphasize that the implementation of any NMDS requires the use of a common language for nursing practice, consistent and complete documentation, and a computerized support application to facilitate the documentation, and the linkage, storage, and retrieval of data. (ANA, 1995b).*

The Nursing Minimum Data Set was the first attempt to standardize the collection of essential uniform nursing data for use across settings and patients groups (ANA, 1995a; ANA, 1995b). The purposes of the NMDS are to:

- Allow the establishment of comparability of nursing across clinical populations, settings, geographic areas, and time;

- Describe nursing care of patients or clients and their families in a variety of settings, both institutional and non-institutional;

- Demonstrate or project trends regarding nursing care that is provided and nursing resources that are allocated to patients or clients according to their health problems and nursing diagnoses;

- Stimulate nursing research through links to the detailed data existing in nursing and other health information systems; and

- Provide data about nursing care to facilitate and influence clinical, administrative, and health policy decision making.

The NMDS includes three broad categories consisting of sixteen groups of data elements categorized as:

(a) *Four nursing care elements*: nursing problem or diagnosis, nursing interventions, nursing outcomes, and intensity of nursing care;

(b) *Five patient or client demographic elements*: personal identification, date of birth, sex, race and culture, and residence;

(c) *Seven service elements*: unique facility or service agency number, unique health record number or chart, unique number of principal registered nurse provider, episode admission or encounter date, discharge or termination date, disposition of patient or chart, and expected payer for most of the bill.

> *Clinical outcomes that result from nursing care rarely occur in isolation. Rather, nursing care occurs within the context of an organized system of nursing care delivery embedded within an organization/network and the broader healthcare delivery system. It is crucial that data that reflect the context within which the care is being delivered be collected and analyzed to answer questions about the effectiveness of clinical nursing intervention strategies. Those questions relate to quality, access, cost, and satisfaction.*

Were NMDSs adopted nationally or worldwide with a system of data collection and processing, the following are the expected benefits for nursing practice:

- Access to comparable minimum nursing care and resources data at local, regional, national, and international levels;

- Enhanced documentation of nursing care provided;

- Incentive to improve methods of costing nursing services;

- Improved data for quality enhancement;

- Stimulus to the development and refinement of nursing information systems;

- Comparative research on nursing care, including research on nursing diagnoses, nursing interventions, nursing-sensitive outcomes, intensity of nursing care, and referral for further nursing services;

- Contribution toward advancement in nursing as a research-based discipline.

The potential of standardized data sets to describe and test nursing science and systems can be enhanced if a synergy can be created among several international communities to identify a common core of elements and their definitions that cross national boundaries. Supported by the collaborative efforts of the International Medical Informatics Association Nursing Informatics Special Interest Group (IMIA-NI SIG) and the International Council for Nurses, specific efforts are underway to create an International Nursing Minimum Data Set (i-NMDS) (Clark and Delaney, 2000).

The Nursing Management Minimum Data Set (NMMDS), co-developed by Delaney and Huber (1996) identifies organizational variables known to be the critical link in determining the effect that nursing diagnoses and interventions have on patient outcomes. The NMMDS focuses on the context of care and serves as a complementary minimum data set to the clinical minimum data set. It includes 17 data elements, structured in three sections:

- *Environment*: type of nursing delivery unit/service; patient/client population; volume of nursing delivery unit/service; nursing delivery unit/service accreditation; decisional population; unit/service complexity; patient/client accessibility; method of care delivery; and complexity of clinical decision making.

- *Nurse Resources*: manager demographic profile; nursing staff and client care support personnel; nursing care staff demographic profile; and nursing care staff satisfaction.

- *Financial Resources*: payer type; reimbursement; nursing delivery unit or service budget; and expenses.

Several actions must be taken once the use of the NMDS is understood as an essential tool in summarizing nursing information and in the facilitation of the evaluation of costs and effectiveness of nursing care:

- *Educate nurses to ensure the quality of nursing data and information in a documentation system;*

- *Create mechanisms to evaluate the content of minimum data sets in a fast and easy way;*

- *Disseminate the idea of minimum data sets national and internationally as a resource to compare nursing intervention and outcomes;*

- *Use the result of minimum data set analyses to influence decision and policy makers.*

Efforts to develop and implement an International Nursing Minimum Data Set (i-NMDS) are being carried out throughout the world.

Examples of national initiatives include those in Australia, Belgium, Canada, Iceland, Korea, Netherlands, Spain, Switzerland, Thailand, United Kingdom, and the United States.

The Australian data set has been constructed for use in community settings. The Canadian data set is mandated federally, while the Belgian data set has been used since 1987. In Spain, extensive work has been done to develop a multi-dimensional data set that includes elements of the NMDS and from DRGs (Diagnostic Related Groups) to support cost analysis and eventually reimbursement for services (ISECS, 2001). Although similarities and differences exist among these data sets in terms of data elements and their definition, all include most of the nursing care elements of the NMDS.

In addition to the numerous NMDS being proposed and the efforts for the definition of an international version (i-NMDS) of NMDS, research still has to be done to test and demonstrate the potential of the established NMDS in describing nursing science and systems. Practicing nurses must realize the importance and value of consistent complete documentation. Leadership is needed to continue to find solutions to issues such as classification taxonomies and the development of comparable languages (Ryan and Delaney, 1995; Clark and Delaney, 2000; Delaney et al., 2000).

Further, attention must be directed to the coordination and linkage of data. There are three aspects of data linkage that demand attention. First, the computer hardware must support database linkage. Secondly, the content of the NMDS must be developed in a way that lends itself to integration with other information. Finally, the ethics of data linkage with respect to patient information, including security, confidentiality, and privacy of data, must be addressed (Hannah et al., 1994).

45

5. Classification Systems in Nursing

Up to now, the nursing profession does not have standardized vocabularies, taxonomies, and classification schemes that could be universally used to represent all elements of nursing practice in all different settings where nursing is exercised. However, nursing classification schemes, taxonomies, and vocabularies are being studied and developed by several researchers throughout the world and this work has given rise to an increasing number of terminologies. These generally take the form of controlled vocabularies.

Because of the controlled vocabulary approach, individual terminologies tend to be tuned to meet the specific requirements of their intended users. To agree on a single, multipurpose terminology is problematic (Simões, 1988; Wright, 1995; Rodrigo, 1997). However, several options for resolving differences between existing terminologies are currently being explored (McCormick et al., 1994; Chute et al., 1996; Henry and Mead, 1997; Campbell et al., 1997; Chute et al., 1998; Campbell et al. 1998; Cimino, 1998; Pascal and Frecon-Valentin, 1998; Hardiker, 2000; ISECS, 2001).

> *Nursing classification systems often aspire to become nursing data standards by offering as a data standard a closed set of nursing concepts in a pre-combined ordering authorized and recognized, where, however, the underlying concept standard remains implicit.*

The European Committee for Standardization Health Informatics Technical Committee (CEN TC251) is developing classification system models to be used by the European Union Member States (CEN, 1997; Ehnfors et al., 1999). Such classification models are conceptually similar to the ones being developed in the United States and recognized by the American Nurses Association (ANA).

Some classification systems are being developed not only to support the five phases of the Nursing Process (*Assessment, Diagnosis, Planning Goals and Interventions, Implementation,* and *Evaluation*) but also to be an integral part of computer-based health record (Grobe, 1996; Henry et al., 1998b; Button et al., 1998; Ceusters, 1999; Chute, 1999; Cimino, 1999; Huff and Carter, 1999; ISO, 1999; Bakken et al., 2000; Beya, 2000). There are classification schemes that involve all phases of the process; others focus on one or more aspects of the Nursing Process, e.g., diagnosis, outcomes, or interventions.

A review of two current systems and their proposed revisions (North American Nursing Diagnosis Association and the International Classification for Nursing Practice), confronted with the features suggested by the Computer-based Patient Record Institute (CPRI) for classification systems appropriate for implementation in computer-based systems, suggests that the evolving versions have atomic and compositional character with sufficient granularity in terms of depth and level of detail (Moen et al., 1999).

Although the most important driving forces for standardization of nursing terminologies are the wish to implement cost measurement and the need for a uniform system as basis for service reimbursement, all taxonomies are, to a great extent, oriented by a clinical and patient-oriented perspective. There is great interest in the creation of a standardized multidimensional classification of nursing diagnoses and interventions that intersect with established classifications of medical diagnoses and interventions based on costs (e.g., Diagnosis Related Groups) and attempts are being made to design such systems (ISECS, 2001).

5.1. The Omaha System - Applications for Community Health Nursing

The Omaha System is a taxonomy designed for the documentation of interdisciplinary practice and data management in community settings. The taxonomy consists of three classification schemes: *Problem Classification Scheme, Intervention Scheme,* and *Problem Rating Scale for Outcomes*. These three components represent an approach to practice, documentation, and information management that is both structured and comprehensive (Martin and Scheet, 1992; Martin and Scheet, 1995; Martin and Norris, 1996).

5.1.1. Problem Classification Scheme

The Problem Classification Scheme is a framework of client-, family-, and community-focused problems amenable to nursing intervention. It is a taxonomy of nursing diagnoses that was developed by community health nurses in extensive research and testing using actual patient data. It provides a comprehensive method for collecting, sorting, classifying, documenting, and analyzing client data for the community nurse, supervisor, and agency administrator. It enables nurses to sort essential from nonessential data objectively and efficiently as well as to identify meaningful patterns in the data.

The classification scheme does not include medical diagnoses, laboratory tests, etiology, and related factors. The Problem Classification Scheme consists of forty-four problems categorized in four domains: *Environmental, Psychosocial, Psychological,* and *Health-related Behaviors.*

Two sets of modifiers are used in conjunction with each problem. When an actual problem modifier is used, a cluster of problem-specific signs and symptoms is used to provide the diagnostic clues to problem identification. The ordering of problems within the domains is based on three principles: (1) terms within each level are stated at the same degree of abstraction – descending from general to problem-specific signs and symptoms; (2) the scheme is comprehensive at the domain and modifier level and incomplete at the level of problems, signs and symptoms, and risk factors; (3) terms are mutually exclusive.

5.1.2. Intervention Scheme

The Intervention Scheme is a systematic arrangement of nursing activities. The intention is to clarify nursing decision and to help nurses and other community care providers to document plans and interventions. The Intervention Scheme is organized in three hierarchical levels:

- Level 1. Categories - used by a community health nurse to develop a plan or document an intervention specific to a client problem representing the final results of the data collection;

- Level 2. Targets - objects of nursing intervention of which the nurse selects one or more to further describe a plan of intervention;

- Level 3. Client-specific information - the detailed portion of a plan or intervention, generated by healthcare provider, designed for client-specific information.

5.1.3. *Problem Rating Scale for Outcomes*

It is designed to measure client progress in relation to specific client problems. Also, it is based on the assumption that the interactions of a community health nurse and a client in relation to a problem affect what client *knows* (knowledge), *does* (behavior), and *is* (status)

- Knowledge: the ability of the client to remember and interpret information;

- Behavior: the observable responses, actions, or activities of the client fit to the occasion or purpose;

- Status: the condition of the client in relation to objective and subjective defining characteristics.

5.2. North American Nursing Diagnoses Association (NANDA)

Since 1970, the NANDA Nursing Diagnoses List has been the predominant listing used by nurses around the world. NANDA defined Nursing Diagnoses as "a clinical judgment about individual, family, or community responses to actual or potential health problems or life processes". Nursing diagnoses provide the basis for the selection of nursing interventions to achieve outcomes for which the nurse is accountable (NANDA, 1993; NANDA, 1999).

Consistent conceptual analysis based in nursing research has been used in the development and refinement of applications to a broad variety of practice environments. Translations to different languages have been done – for experiences in Latin America see Goethe, 1989; Perez et al., 1990; Cruz, 1990a; Cruz, 1990b; Cruz and Cruz, 1991; Jesus, 1992; Cruz, 1992; Dalri, 1993; Rossi and Dalri, 1993; Nobrega, 1994; Zanetti et al., 1994; Jesus, 1995; Robazzi et al., 1995. However, the classification is not universally accepted (Henry et al., 1994; Guirao i Goris et al., 1999).

The classification of nursing diagnosis is based on Human Response Patterns, a list with 128 nursing diagnoses categorized according to nine patterns (ANA, 1995a; ANA, 1998a): *Exchanging, Communicating, Relating, Valuing, Choosing, Moving, Perceiving, Knowing,* and *Feeling.* An extended set of diagnoses, the Nursing Diagnosis Extension Classification (NDEC) has been published, adding another 2,000 diagnoses to the original listing (Clark et al., 2000; Craft-Rosenberg et al., 2000).

5.2.1. *Diagnosis Concepts in NANDA List*

There are three types of nursing diagnosis concepts: *actual nursing diagnoses, at-risk nursing diagnoses, and wellness nursing diagnoses.* Clusters of defining characteristics, signs and symptoms, or clinical cues manifest actual nursing diagnoses. At-risk nursing diagnoses describe human responses that may be developed in vulnerable individuals, families, or communities. Wellness nursing diagnoses describe responses to levels of wellness in individuals, families, or communities. The taxonomy provides a beginning classification scheme, which can be used to categorize and classify nursing diagnostic labels. The rules of classification used for development that were also adopted by several classification system developers are:

- There is no inherent order – one pattern is not considered better than another;

- The level of abstraction determines the level of placement: general to specific, abstract to concrete;

- The diagnosis is classified by considering the definition of the pattern and the diagnosis;

- The placement of the diagnosis is conceptually consistent with the current theoretical views within nursing;

- Categories in brackets were developed by the committee to clarify why certain diagnoses were placed at a specific level or in a specific pattern and from a collaborative effort with the American Nurses Association;

- A numbering system was developed to facilitate computerization of the taxonomy.

The evaluation of cost-effectiveness of NANDA when compared to simple problem listing in risk diagnosis has shown that the former is significantly better (Vazquez et al., 1998).

5.2.2. The NANDA Taxonomy

The new approved NANDA Taxonomy 2 was presented at the Nursing Terminology Summit Conference 2000, hosted by Vanderbilt University (Nashville, Tennessee, USA). This taxonomy comprises six *Axes* and thirteen *Domains*:

Axis 1: The diagnostic concept
Axis 2: Time
Axis 3: Unit of care
Axis 4: Age
Axis 5: Probability
Axis 6: Descriptor

The following table summarizes the domains and respective classes of data involved:

DOMAIN	CLASSES
1. *Health Promotion*	Health awareness, Health management
2. *Nutrition*	Ingestion, Digestion, Absorption, Metabolism, Hydration
3. *Elimination*	Bladder/Kidney, Bowel, Skin, Lungs
4. *Activity/Rest*	Sleep/Rest, Activity/Exercise, Energy field, Cardiovascular pulmonary responses
5. *Perception/ Cognition*	Attention, Orientation, Cognition/Perception, Cognition, Communication
6. *Self-perception*	Self concept, Self-esteem, Body image
7. *Role Relationships*	Caregiver roles, Family relationships, Role performance
8. *Sexuality*	Sexual identity, Sexual function, Reproduction
9. *Coping/Stress Tolerance*	Post-trauma responses, Coping, Neuro-behavioral stress
10. *Life Principles*	Values, Beliefs, Value/Beliefs congruence
11. *Safety/Protection*	Infection, Physical injury, Violence, Environmental hazards, Immune responses, Thermoregulation
12. *Comfort*	Physical comfort, Environmental comfort, Social comfort
13. *Growth/Development*	Growth, Development

5.3. Nursing Interventions Classification (NIC)

The Iowa Nursing Interventions Classification (NIC) is a categorization system of direct care activities performed by nurses, including both direct and indirect care. Nursing Intervention is defined as "any direct care treatment that nurse performs on behalf of a client. These treatment include nurse-initiative treatments resulting from nursing diagnoses, physician-initiated treatments resulting from medical diagnoses, and performance of daily essential functions for the client who cannot do these" (McCloskey and Bulechek, 1992).

The interventions are grouped in 30 classes and 7 domains, which are presented in the table that follows:

DOMAIN	CLASSES
1. Physiological: Basic	Activity and exercise management, Elimination management, Immobility management, ition support, Physical comfort promotion, Self-care facilitation
2. Physiological: Complex	Electrolyte and acid-base management, Drug management, Neurologic management, Perioperative care, Respiratory management, Skin/Wound management, Thermoregulation, Tissue perfusion management
3. Behavioral	Behavior therapy, Cognitive therapy, Communication enhancement, Coping assistance, Patient education, Physiological comfort promotion
4. Safety	Crisis management, Risk management,
5. Family	Childbearing care, Child-rearing care, Lifespan care
6. Health System	Health system mediation, Health system management, Information management
7. Community	Community health promotion, Community risk management

Presently NIC consists of 486 interventions (433 in the second edition, and 336 in the first edition). Each intervention has a label name, definition, and a set of activities that the nurse carries out. The Classification System has three levels of abstraction: *Domain, Classes* and *Intervention List*. In the highest level of abstraction there are seven *Domains*. At the second level of abstraction there are thirty *Classes* of interventions. The third level consists of specific interventions (McCloskey and Bulechek, 1992; McCloskey and Bulechek, 1996; McCloskey and Bulechek, 2000). An example follows:

NIC Level 1 *Domain*   - Physiological: Basic
NIC Level 2 *Class* – Activity and exercise management
NIC Level 3 *Intervention* – Body mechanics promotion
      - Exercise therapy
      - Balance
      - Joint Mobility

The language used is similar to that used by nurses every day to describe the interventions. The classification does not prescribe interventions per diagnoses or patient conditions. Nurses select those interventions that the patient requires and through a paper- or computer-based system link interventions to their corresponding nursing diagnoses and expected outcomes. In addition, a list providing linkages between NANDA nursing diagnoses and NIC Interventions has been developed. This linkage is defined as a relationship between a nursing diagnosis and a nursing intervention that causes them to occur together in order to obtain an outcome or end point of patient problem resolution (ANA, 1995b; Johnson et al., 2001).

5.4. Nursing Outcomes Classification (NOC)

The Nursing Outcomes Classification (NOC) is a comprehensive, standardized classification of patient outcomes developed to evaluate the effects of nursing interventions. An *outcome* is stated as "a variable concept representing an individual, family, or community condition that is measurable along a continuum and responsive to nursing interventions".

NOC outcomes are grouped in a coded taxonomy that organizes the outcomes within a conceptual framework to facilitate locating an outcome. The outcomes are developed for use in all settings and with all patient populations. Since the outcomes describe patient/client status, other disciplines may find them useful for the evaluation of their interventions. The 260 NOC outcomes of the second edition of the Nursing Outcomes Classification are listed in alphabetical order and grouped into twenty-nine classes and seven domains for ease of use.

The seven domains are: Functional Health, Physiologic Health, Psychosocial Health, Health Knowledge & Behavior, Perceived Health, Family Health, and Community Health. Each outcome has a unique code number that facilitates its use in computerized clinical information systems and for the manipulation of data to answer questions about nursing care quality and effectiveness. The classification is continually updated to include new outcomes and to revise older outcomes based on new research or user feedback.

Each outcome has a label name; a definition, a set of indicators that describe specific patient, caregiver, family or community states related to the outcome; a 5-point Likert-type measurement scale; and selected references used in the development of the outcomes. Currently, the taxonomy has seven *Domains* and twenty-none *Classes*.

DOMAIN	CLASSES
1. Functional Health	Energy maintenance, Growth and development, Mobility, Self-care
2. Physiological Health	Cardiopulmonary, Elimination, Fluid and electrolytes, Immune response, Metabolic regulation, Neurocognitive, Nutrition, Therapeutic response, Tissue integrity, Sensory function
3. Psychosocial Health	Psychological wellbeing, Psychosocial adaptation, Self-control, Social interaction
4. Health Knowledge and Behavior	Health behavior, Health beliefs, Health knowledge, Risk control and safety
5. Perceived Health	Health and life quality, Symptom, Status
6. Family Health	Family caregiver status, Family member health status, Family wellbeing
7. Community Health	Community wel-being, Community health protection

Examples of scales of intensity used with the NOC outcomes are: 1 = extremely compromised to 5 = not compromised or 1 = never demonstrated to 5 = consistently demonstrated. Since the outcomes are developed for use in all settings, they can be used across the care continuum to follow patient outcomes throughout an illness episode or over an extended period of care (Johnson and Maas, 1997; Johnson et al., 2000; Johnson et al., 2001).

5.5. Home Healthcare Classification System (HHCC System)

The Home Healthcare Classification (HHCC) System was developed from the Home Care Project conducted by Saba (Saba, 1995a; Saba, 1995b) at Georgetown University School of Nursing. It was designed to develop a method to predict home healthcare needs and resource use for Medicare and elderly populations, including their outcomes of care. The HHCC was designed to assess and document – record and track over time – home health and ambulatory care nursing services. The HHCC System is based on a conceptual framework that uses the six steps of the nursing process to assess patients in a holistic manner.

The HHCC System uses two vocabularies developed by Saba – HHCC of Nursing Diagnoses and HHCC of Nursing Interventions – designed to document, assess, code, and classify home health nursing practice.

5.5.1. HHCC Care Components

The HHCC of Nursing Diagnoses and HHCC of Nursing Interventions vocabularies are classified according to twenty components. They are: *Activity, Bowel Elimination, Cardiac, Cognitive, Coping, Fluid Volume, Health Behavior, Medication, Metabolic, Nutritional, Physical Regulation, Respiratory, Role Relationship, Safety, Self-Care, Self-Concept, Sensory, Skin Integrity, Tissue Perfusion,* and *Urinary Elimination*. Those components are grouped according to four care patterns: *Behavioral, Functional, Physiological,* and *Psychological*.

5.5.2. HHCC of Nursing Diagnoses

The HHCC of Nursing Diagnoses consists of 145 nursing diagnoses, of which 50 are major nursing diagnostic categories (represented by a two-digit code) and 95 are subcategories (three-digit codes). The HHCC of Nursing Diagnoses uses the definition put forth by the North American Nursing Diagnoses Association (NANDA) and consists of empirically developed home health nursing diagnostic labels. Further, each nursing diagnostic label is structured as a noun phrase instead of a verb phrase and is coded with one of three modifiers representing one expected outcome or goal of the care as determined by the planned interventions.

The HHCC System makes it possible not only to assess and document, but also to code, index, link, and map the six steps of the nursing process and its two vocabularies – the HHCC of Nursing Diagnoses and HHCC of Nursing Interventions. This innovative system, moreover, provides the coding strategy for computer-based patient record, which can be used to generate the evidence needed to track the care process across time, settings, and geographic locations.

The HHCC System is used to document and track evidence-based nursing practice. It provides the evidence needed to: (a) improve efficiency of assessing and documenting care; (b) establish patterns for care; (c) develop a cost-effective method for evaluating quality and outcomes of care; and (d) develop a costing method for reimbursement and payment.

The HHCC of Nursing Diagnoses and HHCC of Nursing Interventions vocabularies are classified according to twenty *Care Components* grouped by the four *Care Patterns.*

CARE PATTERNS	CARE COMPONENTS
1. Behavioral	Health behavior, Medications, Safety
2. Functional	Activity, Fluid volume, Nutrition, Self-care, Sensory
3. Physiological	Bowel elimination, Cardiac, Metabolic, Physical Regulation, Respiratory, Skin integrity, Tissue perfusion, Urinary elimination
4. Psychological	Cognitive, Coping, Role relationship, Self-concept

5.5.3. *HHCC Nursing Diagnosis Outcomes*

The HHCC of Nursing Diagnoses also uses a modifier to determine the expected outcome goal for each nursing diagnosis. However, because a specific outcome measure is determined to be the goal of home healthcare, it is also considered to be another facet of the nursing diagnosis label, and used to evaluate the actual outcome of the care. As a result, the three modifiers consisting of three codes listed below form another data dictionary.

In summary, the modifiers in this data dictionary are used to identify an expected outcome or goal for each identified nursing diagnosis as well as used to evaluate the actual outcome of the care provided. They are coded as: 1 = Improved; 2 = Stabilized; and 3 = Deteriorated.

5.5.4.   HHCC of Nursing Interventions

The HHCC of Nursing Interventions consists of 160 nursing interventions, of which 60 labels are major nursing intervention categories (two-digit codes) and 100 are subcategories (three-digit codes). A Nursing Intervention is defined as a single nursing service, treatment, procedure, or activity and designed as a response to a diagnosis. It encompasses the need to obtain evidence of the outcome (medical or nursing) for which a nurse is responsible. Further, each nursing intervention item is coded with one of four modifiers representing type of nursing intervention action provided during a specific nursing care service.

5.5.5.   HHCC Type of Nursing Intervention

The HHCC of Nursing Interventions also uses a modifier to identify the type of nursing intervention action provided during a specific care service. Each of the four modifiers represents a different time and/or cost factor. In summary, these four modifiers expand the number of Nursing Interventions from 160 to 640 possible actions. The four codes are:

1 = Access / Monitor
2 = Direct Care / Perform
3 = Teach / Supervise
4 = Manage / Refer

5.5.6.   Coding Strategy

The two HHCC vocabularies and their modifiers are coded according to rules that are similar to the Tenth Revision of the International Classification of Diseases (ICD-10). HHCC codes consists of a five-character alphanumeric sequence represented as follows:

- Starting at the leftmost character, the first position is an alphabetic character representing the Care Component;

- The second and third positions together represent a two-digit code indicating the major (diagnostic or intervention) category;

- Following a decimal point is the fourth position, which is a one-digit code for diagnostic or intervention subcategory, if it exists;

- The digit in the fifth position is a one-digit code representing the modifier (expected /actual outcome or type intervention action).

5.6. International Classification for Nursing Practice (ICNP)

The International Council of Nursing (ICN) is composed of 126 members representing 105 national nursing associations and 21 WHO Nursing Collaborating Centers. As part of its commitment to advance nursing throughout the world, the ICN has initiated a long-term project to develop an International Classification for Nursing Practice (ICNP).

There are many compelling reasons to develop a single system, the foremost being the evident need to clarify and to improve nursing knowledge, in order to improve quality in nursing care (Clark, 1992; Henry et al., 1998a; Mortensen, 1999). Also, a universal classification advances the interest in recording nursing contribution to healthcare and contributes to better use of the ubiquitous computerization of processes and routines taking place in the health sector.

The overall goals of such a classification are to support the processes of nursing practice and to advance the knowledge necessary for cost-effective delivery of quality nursing care (Ehnfors, 1999; Nielsen and Mortensen, 1999). Those goals are to be achieved by the establishment of a common language about nursing practice capable of describing nursing care; permitting comparison of nursing data; able to demonstrate or project tendencies; and capable of stimulating nursing research. (ICN, 1993; ICN, 1996; ICN 1999).

In 1993, a draft of the classification scheme was proposed. This draft, called ICNP – International Classification of Nursing Practice – included not only the four classification schemes recognized by the committee led by the American Nursing Association but also other schemes developed internationally. The intention of ICNP is to obtain a world representative sample to construct a comprehensive classification scheme, eventually to be used by nurses all over the world.

The framework for the classification includes three elements: (1) nursing problems (diagnoses), (2) nursing interventions (actions), and (3) nursing outcomes. Each of the elements is alphabetized and compared to terms used in member countries. The International Classification for Nursing Practice, alpha version, was published in 1996. It consists of two sections: *nursing phenomena* and *nursing interventions*.

The classification of nursing phenomena and nursing interventions serves as a guide to exact definitions of concepts, because a classification by generic relationships between concepts is serviceable in offering definitions by genus and species (Mortensen, 1996; Nielsen 1997; Nielsen and Mortensen, 1997a; Nielsen and Mortensen, 1997b). Problems were found in attempts to map the terms of ICNP alpha version to nursing problem lists for specific application areas (Gutierrez et al., 1999).

The term "nursing phenomena" was elected because it is a neutral term toward any existing particular framework or nursing care model. It also appears adequate, since its literal meaning is "what can be observed". Nursing phenomena are defined as factors influencing health status with the defining characteristic that they are what nurses diagnose. The naming of nursing phenomena and their representation in a standardized manner suitable for encoding in computer-based systems and electronic medical records present a challenge for the nursing profession. The ICNP, alpha version, comprises a list of 297 terms to describe nursing phenomena. It has a mono-axial structure, focused on nursing practice (Nielsen and Mortensen, 1996; Nielsen, 1996).

"Nursing interventions" are defined as types of actions taken by nurses in response to nursing phenomena. The ICNP, alpha version, also includes the Nursing Interventions classification, which has a multi-axial structure.

The axes are:

- Actions types in nursing practice;

- Object types in nursing practice;

- Types of generating activities in nursing practice;

- Means in nursing practice;

- Anatomical sites in nursing practice;

- Time/Place in nursing practice.

In June 1999, the beta version of the International Classification for Nursing Practice was released by ICN (Nielsen, 1999a; Nielsen 1999b). The components are: *Nursing Phenomena (problems, needs, and diagnoses); Nursing Actions (interventions),* and *Nursing Outcomes.* The beta version supports a broad definition of health and it is expanded to include primary healthcare, including community-based nursing concepts. The nursing phenomena is now a multi-axial classification with eight axes: *Focus of Nursing Practice, Judgement, Frequency, Duration, Body Site, Laterality, Distribution,* and *Likelihood.* The Action (formerly name "nursing intervention") Classification continues to be a multi-axial structure in which the terms can be combined to establish the entire phrase that will prescribe the nursing treatment. The axes are: *Action Type, Target, Means, Time, Location, Topology, Routes,* and *Beneficiary.*

6.   Nursing Informatics

The International Medical Informatics Association - Nursing Informatics (IMIA-NI) defines Nursing Informatics as: *"... the integration of nursing, its information, and information management with information processing and communication technologies, to support the health of people world wide."*

One major effort in Nursing Informatics is to specify clinical information system requirements which include nurses' needs for information processing to support their practice, including specifications for data and systems standards (Zielstorff et al., 1993; Hannah et al., 1994; Barnett, 1995; Saba and McCormick, 1996; Button et al., 1998; PAHO, 1999a; Mayes, 2000; WHO, 2000; Saba and McCormick, 2001).

An information system consists of people, information, procedures, hardware, and software. Working together, they accomplish a set of specific functions. Ideally, people, information system, and work processes operate in concert to maximize the benefits of human and technology capacities. For these benefits to happen, reviewing, rethinking, and changing existing work flows, routines, and current practices are required. Likewise, it is imperative to fully understand nursing information needs and explicitly communicate these needs to system developers, so that automated systems can be developed that satisfy the expectations of the final users and truly serve practice. Implementation of information systems into the workplace produces many predictable and unpredictable ("unintended consequences") impacts on the work environment as well as on the workers.

Whether using a manual or an automated information system to manage data, it is imperative that retrieval of required data can be achieved in a fast and uncomplicated way. In the healthcare sector a single database has limited usage and value, whereas several linked and integrated databases within one or more information systems have the capacity to add value by reducing the time required to generate complex information needed to support clinical and administrative decision making (Yoshioca et al., 1994)

Distributed databases of increasing complexity and variety of data contents will be increasingly used by the health sector. Such databases are required because of the size and variety of functions of health organizations along with the need for multi-site access to longitudinal patient records, continuity of care over the lifetime of clients, and the management requirements of insurers, payers, and regulators. However, accessibility and implementation of data retrieval and analysis mechanisms operating on distributed databases are dependent upon an appropriate and reliable telecommunications infrastructure and systems functioning under technical standards and protocols.

6.1. Information Technology and the Nursing Profession

Most nurses continue to have difficulties in embracing information technologies in support of their practice. Furthermore, it continues to be a challenge for nurses to obtain appropriate education in informatics both in the undergraduate and graduate curricula and as a component of postgraduate specialist courses (Soto et al., 1992; Scochi et al., 1993).

When a computerized information system is introduced nurses are immediately confronted with new technologies, jargon, and a diverse system of beliefs, values, and assumptions about their professional work. This impact of these systems is particularly significant in developing countries (Scochi et al., 1991; Luis et al., 1992; Evora, 1993)

There is a widespread concern among nurses that nursing services will become depersonalized and that patient and nurses will become appendages to computers. Only recently, with the development of new devices (portable computers, wireless communication, bedside terminals) research has been done to assess nursing expectations, concerns, and willingness to re-conceptualize traditional tasks for adaptation to the growing computer capabilities and variety of interface equipment. Because nurses comprise the majority of the end-users, they should be appropriately consulted. Health professionals may resist using a computer for a variety of reasons. They may manifest opposition in ways that range from passive defiance to outright sabotage of the system.

> *Competence in using a variety of information and telecommunications technologies, information research skills, and higher-order thinking skills are required to function adequately in the 21st century. More specifically, we all require the ability to find, select, retrieve, decode, critically evaluate, and use information to create knowledge and insight. Another requirement is the ability to communicate this knowledge and insight to others through the use of a variety of technologies. This is especially true in the knowledge-intensive health industry. Educational institutions must accept this challenge and prepare health professionals for a lifetime of reskilling, redirection, and reorganization. A knowledge economy requires people who are independent and lifelong learners, able to work in teams and communicate effectively.*

Nursing informatics expertise is essential to ensure that nurses involved in projects effectively interact with systems professionals and contribute to the design of applications. Such expertise is also required in the identification of clinical, management, and community data required to support decision making and knowledge building.

6.2. Computerized Nursing Information Systems

The establishment and operation of an information function component in the context of organizations involve the development and management of three interrelated areas (PAHO, 1999a): *Information Systems (IS), Information Technology (IT),* and *Information Management (IM).*

- *Information Systems (IS)* — Represented by the collection of technical tasks with the objective of ascertaining the demand, contents, data input and information output required, and the data-related flows and routines needed for the construction of the organization's application portfolio. Information Systems are, therefore, basically concerned with "what" is required (demand issues).

- *Information Technology (IT)* — Represented by the collection of technical knowledge and tasks with the objective of satisfying the demand for applications. It involves creating, managing, and supplying the technological resources (hardware, software, and communications) necessary for the development and operation of the applications portfolio of an organization; it is concerned with "how" what is required can be delivered (supply issues).

- *Information Management (IM)* — Represented by the strategic organization-wide involvement of four components: data, information systems, information technology, and information personnel. It comprises the administrative operation and control of implemented systems, procurement, contracting of products and services, systems security, legal and ethical issues, and the all-important education and training of users at all levels.

> *Nursing information systems, to be useful, must allow for a wide scope of health data. To be useful, information systems must capture and process health and health-related data of broad diversity, scope, and level of detail. At all levels, the greatest need remains the establishment of information systems that capture and process data originating from the continuum of care and enable the establishment of longitudinal individual patient records from which data and information recovery can be done from three perspectives: patient-oriented, problem-oriented, and procedure-oriented.*

Information Technology (IT), in a more strict sense, is a machine-based technology that actively processes data and information. IT is just one of a set of information-related technologies that share some characteristics. The definition, however, does not separate active information processing from other technologies and media, such as the telephone and television, and from other information-handling activities not based in digital or computerized resources.

The identification of nursing data needs and the need for nursing concept systems or terminologies, also known as classification systems, can both be seen as the first step indicating the user requirements as stated by the profession of nursing. In a second step towards computerization these user requirements will be analyzed by informaticians, resulting in the design of conceptual models, i.e., simplified verbal, graphical, mathematical, or logical representations of a domain from a certain point of view. An analysis of the nursing data requirements will result in a nursing data model describing structural features related to the organization of nursing data in computerized clinical databases or an information processing system.

The process of developing computerized healthcare information systems, including computerized nursing information systems, involves the sequential successful execution of nine components (Figure 4) related to the development, deployment, and operation of information systems and technology:

- *Plan*
- *Prepare*
- *Procure*
- *Test*
- *Implement*
- *Operate*
- *Maintain*
- *Measure Success*
- *Improve*

Figure 4. Dynamics of the Process of Developing and Operating IS&T

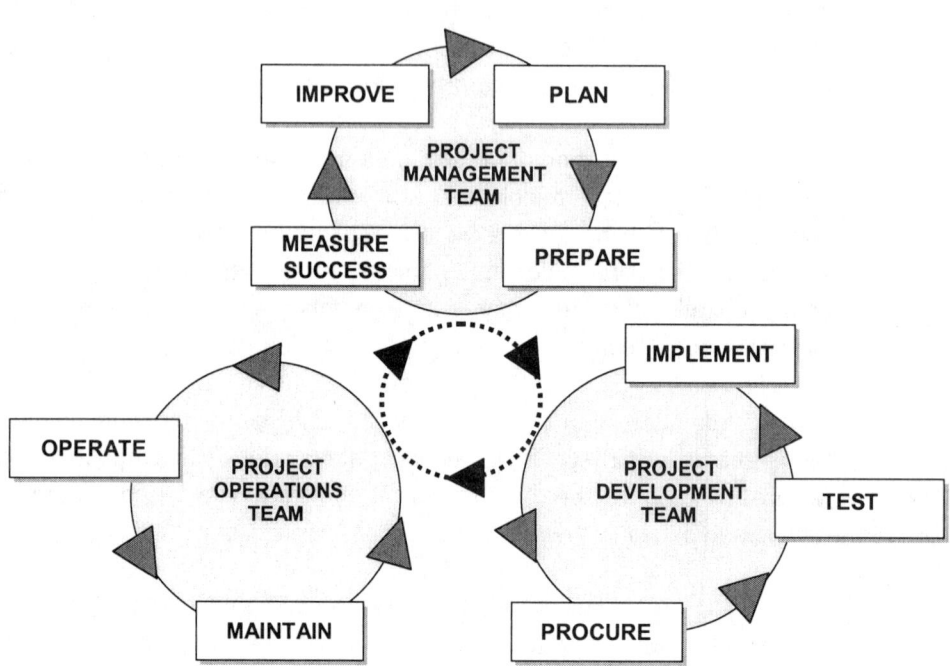

Source: PAHO, 1999a

The most important strategic issues in information systems are related to technology and data standards. Data processing, technical, and electronic standards are essential if equipment is to be able to interconnect. Data definitions and terminologies will be essential if health professionals are to communicate. Specific technical components such as the recording and transmission of images have their own international standards. Requirements for statistical and other analyses to be passed upwards to support informed decision making must be compatible and follow specific standard definitions and conform to country-specific settings.

A prerequisite for the development of nursing computerized systems and electronic patient records is:

- The representation of concepts; functions; nomenclatures; description of signs, symptoms, interventions, and outcomes; and related data such as patient classification, medications, insurance eligibility, etc. and

- The relationships of the above elements in a structured format, amenable to translation into a computer set of instructions and reference tables. The definition of this logical model is accomplished by the careful analysis of the categorical structures and the terminology model that will be used to describe nursing concepts. The logical model will be used as the basis for developing executable computer programs that support the use of both nursing minimum data sets and nursing concept systems or terminologies.

6.3. Standards in Information Systems and Technology

The core concept in open systems is the use of standards. Without easy, reliable, approved ways to connect the necessary components, open systems cannot work.

> *One of the characteristics of health data transmission applications is the integration of technologies, information, and communication systems. The role of standards is well established and founded on the need to avoid market fragmentation, proliferation of incompatible applications, the high costs of developing individual solutions, maintenance problems, and the barriers to achieving the operative integration of different and isolated systems. The coordination and adoption of common standards for users, manufacturers, and service providers foster the production of more cost-effective and stable solutions.*

Within the healthcare industry there are a number of categories of information that each have separate standards (PAHO, 1999a). They are listed here, along with a brief description of the category, and applicable examples of well-known standards:

- *Identifier Standards* - These are themselves subdivided into patient, provider, site-of-care, and product. Not surprisingly, those systems are not universally accepted.

- *Communications (Message Format) Standards* Although the standards in this area are still in various stages of development, they are generally more mature than those of the other groups.

- *Content and Structure Standards* - Work in this area is primarily directed at developing standards for the design of the Computer-based Patient Record.

- *Clinical Data Representations (Codes)* - These are widely used to document diagnoses and procedures. There are over 150 known coding systems, such as the International Classification of Diseases (ICD) system, promoted by the World Health Organization. The American Medical Association (AMA) promotes the Current Procedural Terminology (CPT) coding system in the United States. Another common standard for medical terms is the Systematized Nomenclature of Human and Veterinary Medicine (SNOMED). It has eleven separate axes for categorizing semantic relationships among medical terms. Laboratory Observation Identifier Names and Codes (LOINC) have been developed to create universal test codes for laboratory results and observation messages.

- *Confidentiality, Data Security, and Authentication* - The development of both the Computer-based Patient Record and Healthcare Networks has spurred the need for more definitive confidentiality, data security, and authentication guidelines and standards. Numerous activities are underway to address these issues.

- *Quality Indicators, Data Sets, and Guidelines* - Although there is not an accredited standard to measure healthcare quality, there are several quality indicators, data sets, and guidelines that are gaining acceptance. In the United States examples are: the American Nurses Association (ANA) Quality Indicators and the Health Plan Employer Data and Information Set (HEDIS), the latter developed with the support of the National Committee for Quality Assurance (NCQA). It identifies data to support performance measurement in the areas of quality, access and patient satisfaction, membership and utilization, and finance.

- *International Standards* - The International Standards Organization (ISO) is a worldwide federation of national standards organizations. It has 90 member countries. The purpose of ISO is to promote the development of standardization and related activities in the world. To this end there are many organizations, committees, and subgroups which promote the evolution of healthcare standards worldwide.

- *Nursing Standards* - The American Nursing Association Nursing Information and Data Set Evaluation Center (NIDSEC) is an important professional resource for standards (ANA, 1997). Specific standards for data set and information systems that support nursing practice have been developed; they designate requirements for nomenclature, clinical linkages among nursing diagnoses, interventions, outcomes, etc; nursing data repositories; and information system, administration, and decision support. Terminologies for the representation of nursing concepts, organizations focused on standards development, and the Nursing Management Minimum Data Set (NMMDS) are outlined in detail in Appendices 1 and 2, at the end of this document.

From a healthcare standards perspective, the area of standards is in constant flux. One must be attentive to the evolution of the recommendations of the international and national technical agencies and professional organizations that work on standards research. The knowledgeable healthcare executive will do well to stay current on healthcare standards development. In addition, vendors demonstrating present and future commitment to standards are those most likely to survive in the very competitive healthcare IS&T marketplace, and should be given top consideration by healthcare enterprises in the process of systems selection (PAHO, 1999a).

6.4. User Interface

Nurses' acceptance of a clinical computer-based system directly influences the system's ease of operation and user level of computer and information literacy. Format of data presentation and navigation instructions and sequencing of data entry or retrieval routines must be designed in a way that is meaningful to the nurse and appropriate to the characteristics of the professional work environment.

Nursing information systems involve large volumes of data and great level of detail. They must accommodate a variety of data capture methods such as barcode readers, touch screens, light pens, mouse, voice recognition, and typing. Data entry must be no more time consuming than manual methods for entering comparable data. Where possible data entry should be less time consuming when a computerized system is used.

The user interface design should follow established principles because it has an enormous impact on user training, ongoing efficiency, and staff productivity as well as the system's ability to assist with clinical decision making. Connections to other internal or external systems should appear "seamless" to the user. The latter is achieved via the adoption of technical and terminology standards. The development, adoption, and usage of messaging standards that enable the transfer of data from one system to another is described in a later section. The following table provides a summary of interface design principles.

Design Principles in Computer Systems User Interfaces

USABILITY PRINCIPLES FOR USER INTERFACES	
Simple and natural dialogue	Dialogues should not contain information that is irrelevant or rarely needed. Every extra unit of information in a dialogue competes with the relevant units of information and diminishes their relative visibility. All information should appear in a natural and logical order.
Speak the user's language	The dialogue should be expressed clearly in words, phrases, and concepts familiar to the user, rather than in system-oriented terms.
Minimize the user's memory load	The user should not have to remember information from one part of the dialogue to another. Instructions for use of the system should be visible or easily retrievable whenever appropriate.
Consistency	Users should not have to wonder whether words, situations, and actions mean the same thing.
Provide feedback	The system should always keep users informed about what is going on through appropriate feedback within reasonable time.
Provide clearly marked exits	Users often choose system functions by mistake and will need a clearly marked 'emergency exit' to leave the unwanted state without having to go through an extended dialogue.
Provide shortcuts	Clever shortcuts – unseen by the novice user – may often speed up the interaction for the expert user such that the system caters to both inexperienced and experienced users.
Good error messages	Error messages should be expressed in plain language (no codes), precisely indicate the problem, and constructively suggest a solution.
Prevent errors	Even better than good error messages is a careful design that prevents a problem from occurring in the first place.

Source: Nielsen J. Traditional dialogue design applied to modern user interfaces. Communications of the Association for Computing Machinery 33 1993; (10):109-118 (as published in Zielstorff RD, Hudgings CI, Grobe SJ, and the National Commission on Nursing Implementation Project (NCNIP) Taskforce on Nursing Information Systems. Next-Generation Nursing Information Systems: Essential Characteristics for Practice. American Nurses Association, Washington D.C.; 1993.

6.5. Security, Privacy, and Confidentiality

Security refers to the protection of an information system, including the equipment or computer and the stored data, against deliberate or accidental access, data integrity loss, and data modification, theft, or destruction by an individuals or physical elements. Security involves protecting not only the hardware, but also the information and supporting software from illegal access, fraud, and illicit use.

Security includes physical security, communication security, and data security. Physical security refers to physical threats (e.g., fire, flood, and theft) and deliberate destructive acts. Communication security refers to data protection over telecommunication devices. Protection of data during online transmission is particularly difficult to ensure. Several different actions and devices such as firewalls and encrypting the data are being used to protect the data being transmitted from illegal access and to maintain data integrity (Silberg et al., 1997; Impicciatore et al., 1997; Eng and Gustfson, 1999; Internet Healthcare Coalition, 2000).

Privacy is the ability to control the disclosure and use of information about a patient. Privacy in a computer-based information system assures the patients that their data are protected against improper access and misuse. Federal laws are being mandated to guarantee the public right to privacy and confidentiality of their health data when amassed in national information systems (IITF, 1995; Grenade, 1996; Goodman, 1998; Stanberry, 1998/99; European Union, 1999; Schanz, 1999; Rodrigues, 2000).

Confidentiality is the expectation by a patient that the information provided to an authorized user will not be disclosed. Confidentiality is an ethical obligation that health professionals are bound to honor. Nurses must safeguard the patient's right to privacy by protecting their information in a confidential manner.

Nurses are particularly concerned with the security, privacy, and confidentiality of patient information. There is a common misconception that the paper-based patient records are safer on the nurses' station than as an electronic record in a computer storage device and that the control over privacy and confidentiality is somewhat lost when the patient records are integrated in a computer-based information systems. However, with proper procedures, policies, accreditation requirements, and legislation, computer-based information system standards can provide better privacy and confidentiality of the patient information than that afforded by traditional paper records (Bukovich, 2001).

> *Issues related to security, privacy, and confidentiality include: the high sensitivity of personal data and the damage that its use may bring to individuals; the conflicting demands brought forth by multi-professional access to personally identified data, administrative needs, and access by external stakeholders (e.g., insurance, regulators); the growing trend in remote archiving of medical records; the fact that too many safety barriers interfere with professional work; and the need to balance between individual rights and collective interests (e.g., public health, research). Security is needed to protect privacy and confidentiality, but security implementation measures may interfere with privacy (Council of Europe, 1995; Hodge et al., 1999; UNESCO, 1999; Rodrigues, 2000a).*

Data security risk is very high in health organizations because of the distributed nature of authority and documentation. Sophisticated data protection tools are readily available and can be used for the secure communication of data over public networks. However, opportunity and timeliness of access is an overwhelming requirement for health records, limiting the use of encryption and complex protection schemes for data in use (e.g., a hospitalized patient undergoing treatment). It is important to note that most security violations are not intentional but related to human operational errors and that the most serious infringements are internal to the organization.

Privacy may be difficult to implement due to the multi-professional nature of healthcare and the need for identified personal data by administrative personnel. Anonymous clinical information has no value in individual care but, in some instances, patients may be incapable to authorize access or disclosure of personal data. In sectors were security and confidentiality are essential (e.g., military), it is far better to have data lost than disclosed – the opposite is true for personal data, the risk of disclosure must be accepted in life-threatening situations.

6.6. Management of Change

Nurses play an important role and can positively influence the implementation of a computer-based system using nursing terminologies. To achieve this goal, the implementation of data standards requires change management, and training and education expertise. Change in a pattern of practice or action will occur only as the nurses involved are convinced to change their normal orientations to their old patterns. Change in normative orientation involves changes in attitudes, values, skills, and relationships and not just changes in knowledge, information, or intellectual rationale for action and practice (Hannah et al., 1994).

> *Understanding change theory and its applications is critical to successful implementation of the nursing information system (data) standards. Successful change can be accomplished only by addressing both cognitive and affective components of the nurse's behavior. Education promoting knowledge (cognitive) and concepts relating to attitudes (affective) should be used to promote the desired change.*

According to Ball and Snelbecker (1982), in the past there were several reasons why healthcare professionals, including nurses, were resistant to change toward using technology incorporating information system standards. Amongst them: oversell of systems by vendors, unrealistic expectations of the capabilities of the system, changes in traditional procedures, insufficient involvement of nurses or health providers in the design of systems, and fear of the unknown changes being introduced. Although some of those constraints have eased, others remain, particularly the still limited involvement of nurses in systems specification.

One of the classic theories of change (Lewin, 1969) suggests that behavior in an institutional setting is not a static habit or pattern. Instead change occurs in the context of a balance of forces working in opposite directions within the social-psychological space of the institution. There are three stages in achieving a behavior change according to Lewin: unfreezing the existing equilibrium, movement toward a new equilibrium, and refreezing the new equilibrium. To begin to unfreeze the equilibrium one can: increase the number of driving forces, decrease the number of resisting forces, or a combination of these.

Nurses must be aware of which forces are driving them to a certain goal and which forces are resisting movement toward the goal. Working toward finding a midpoint where the best outcome can occur, nurses need to cope with the resisting forces within the profession so that the result is a stable, predictable, rational approach to improving the quality of nursing practice and the quality of patient care (Hannah et al., 1994).

Strategies used to manage change in nursing and other healthcare professionals should consider the following:

- Involve nurses, users, other health personnel from all departments in the design, development, and testing of information system applications;

- Designate a nurse to coordinate the implementation process within the nursing department;

- Establish a user's committee to introduce change by involving the key players;

- Identify consultants and other resource people who are available during this process;

- Develop a training program to address the "why" or rationale for the system as well as the "advantages" and "disadvantages" of the system;

- Use nursing informatics experts to educate and train the nurse users;

- Provide training prior to and during the implementation phase;

- Provide continuous user support in the operational (production) phase;

- Ensure security, privacy, and confidentiality.

6.7. NUREC: An Example of a Computerized Electronic Nursing Record System for Inpatient Care

The NUREC computerized nursing record application was developed by Gasser and Assimacopoulos at the Unité d'Information Médico-Economique, Hôpitaux Universitaires de Genève Belle-Idée, Chêne-Bourg, Genève in collaboration with the European Committee for Standardization (CEN) and the Danish Institute for Health and Nursing Research/WHO Collaborating Center for Nursing and Midwifery (DIHNR). NUREC runs under the Windows operating system for microcomputers and was developed using the object-oriented programming language Delphi 4 and Paradox 5/7 as the database management system.

NUREC was conceived as an easily implemented electronic record based on the Nursing Process general problem-solving strategy, using the International Classification of Nursing Procedures (ICNP) as a general framework for the description of nursing care. It has been designed as a support to the problem solving strategy used by nurses in their daily practice and demonstrates the feasibility and benefit of computer-supported nursing care. NUREC is built in three modules: a *nomenclature server*, a *nursing care process manager*, and a *care plan manager*.

6.7.1. Modules

The *nomenclature server* module is a browser for the ICNP. It is designed to allow care managers to generate a thesaurus of pre-coded expressions within the ICNP axes and to define links between expression of the thesaurus.

The *nursing care process manager* module four-column display is where the nursing problems, expected outcome, nursing action, and progress notes are recorded. Thesaurus expression (pre-coded expressions from the nomenclature server) are used to describe nursing problems and expected outcome of care actions. Each data item, namely each paragraph in the columns, is composed of a title, a free text description, and specific attributes for handling by the care plan manager or by other browsing functions. Multiple links between each data item allow the user to describe semantic association of problems with other problems, with expected outcomes, care actions, and progress notes.

The *care plan manager* module is where the results of care actions defined in the care process manager module are recorded. It allows the recording of hourly or daily actions planed for a patient, a selected group of patients, or a ward. It can be used by nurses to plan their work, to validate the care effectively provided, and to record direct observations made during care delivery activities.

6.7.2. Functionalities

System Configuration – once the application is installed, the user or users with supervisory rights to the system populate the basic tables (nursing personnel data, data dictionaries, user-interface language), manage user rights (three levels of access are permitted: general user, administrator, and supervisor), enter basic data particular to each institution such as departments, patient units, rooms, and beds (establishment management), draw a graphical representation of each department or unit (map manager), and define technical aspects of the system operation (shutdown conditions and screen resolution).

Thesaurus – this function, accessible only to system supervisors, allows the creation of a structure of database dictionaries containing pre-coded expressions used by the nursing care process manager module. Examples of data sets represented in dictionaries are: health problems, causes, signs, symptoms, goals, and interventions. Each dictionary is organized as a hierarchical tree. Links between items of different dictionaries (e.g., causes with signs) can be created. Selection of a linked item automatically displays the other items to which it is associated.

Security and Confidentiality – three levels of user access are possible, and the individual user is required to use a password. Access to data of care units is limited to the unit or units to which the user is assigned. Read-only or read/write levels of access are also possible.

Admission, Transfer, and Discharge – each inpatient (ward) unit is graphically represented in the main window of the program. Admission of new or return patients, entry of admission data, transfer between units, and institutional discharge are handled by a number of screens (Figures 5, 6, and 7).

Patient Data – authorized users can read, enter, or modify patient data in the following functions: administrative (identification, bed occupied, transfers, discharge, scheduling), clinical documentation (patient record and vital signs), nursing evaluation (problem assessment with corresponding signs and symptoms and identified causes), intervention planning (selection of appropriate intervention (Figures 8, 9, 10, and 11).

Figure 5. The Main User Interface Screen of NUREC

At the top of the screen, information about the present user and ward are displayed. Buttons for different functions permit the user to navigate the application according to the user level of access (privileges) set by the systems administration. Each patient room is represented and the occupied beds are tagged with the corresponding patient name.

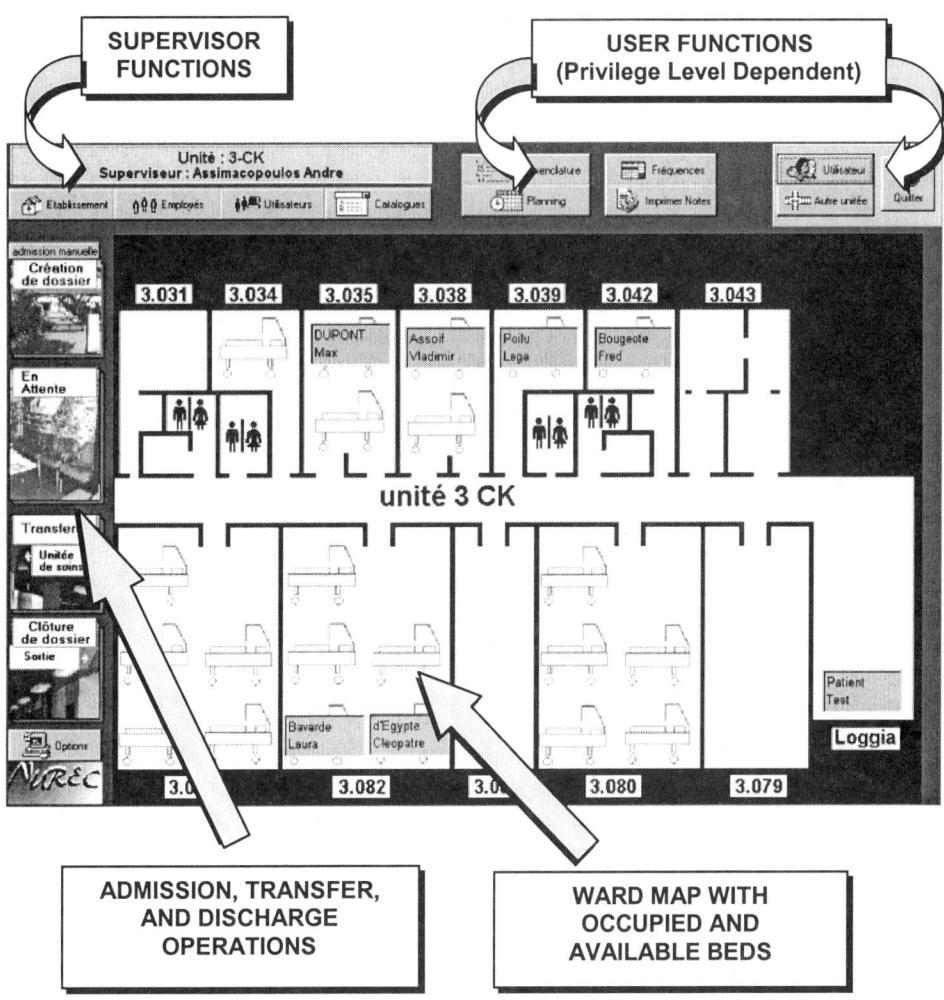

SUPERVISOR FUNCTIONS

USER FUNCTIONS (Privilege Level Dependent)

ADMISSION, TRANSFER, AND DISCHARGE OPERATIONS

WARD MAP WITH OCCUPIED AND AVAILABLE BEDS

Figure 6. Patient Admission Screens

*Patients can be admitted to the ward by selecting an already-
existing record (from a previous admission) or by creating a new
computer database record.*

New Record...

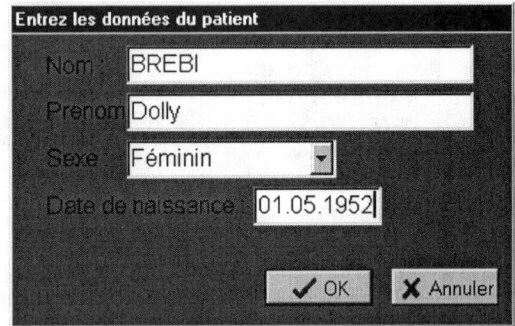

Searching in the Database for a Previous Record...

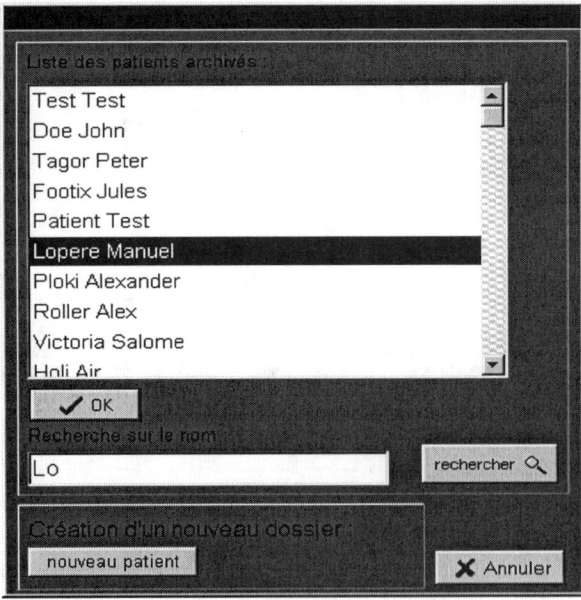

Figure 7. Admission Data

For each patient admission event, data are entered in the corresponding record, including responsible physician, referring institution, reason for admission, type of admission, allergies, and other important patient data and comments in free text.

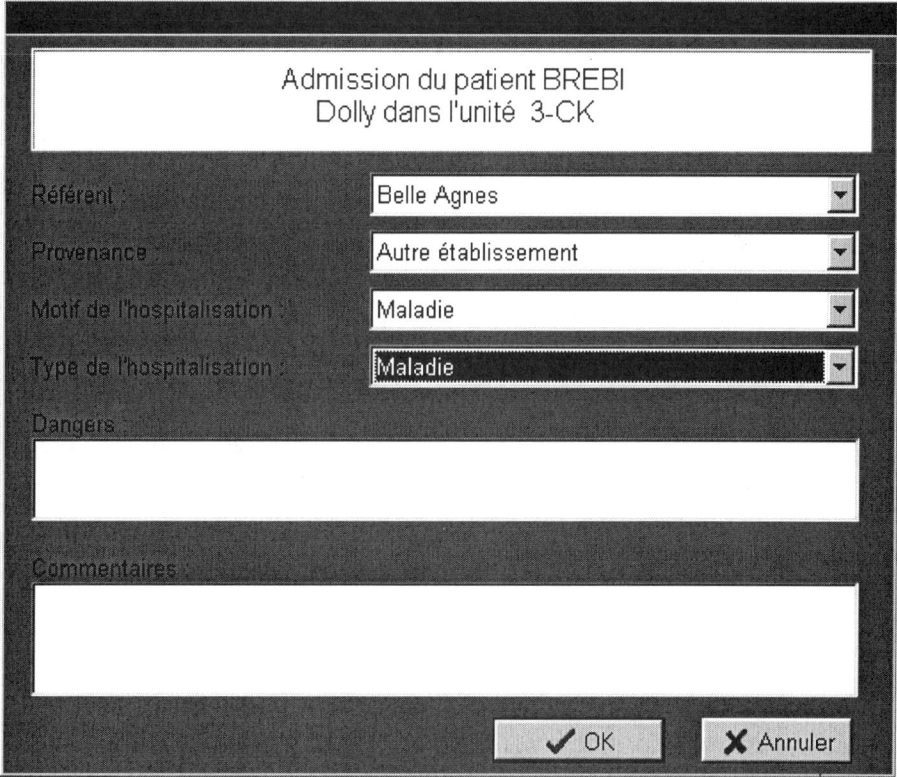

Figure 8. Patient Administrative Data

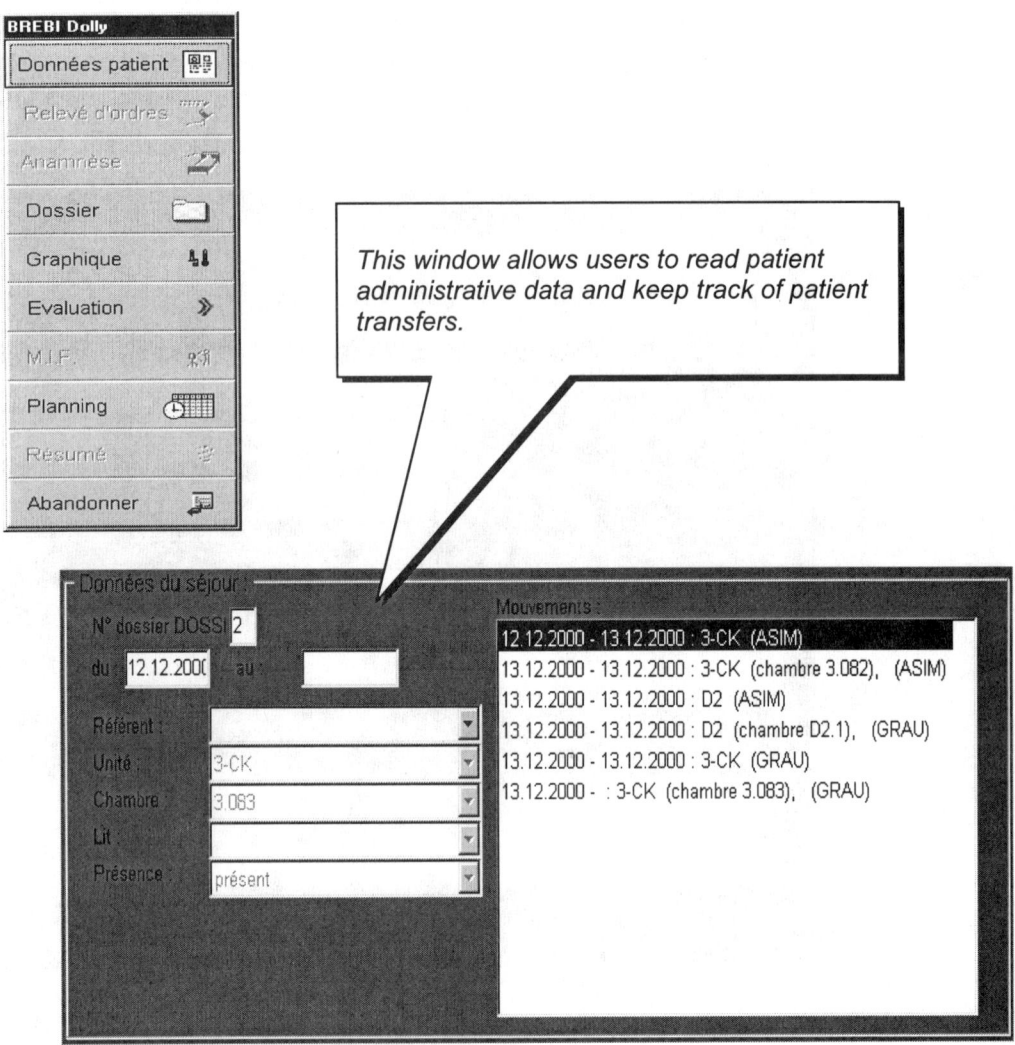

This window allows users to read patient administrative data and keep track of patient transfers.

Figure 9. Patient Clinical Data

Nursing management functions are handled via a four-column electronic form that allows data entry for health problems, nursing care goals, interventions, and progress notes.

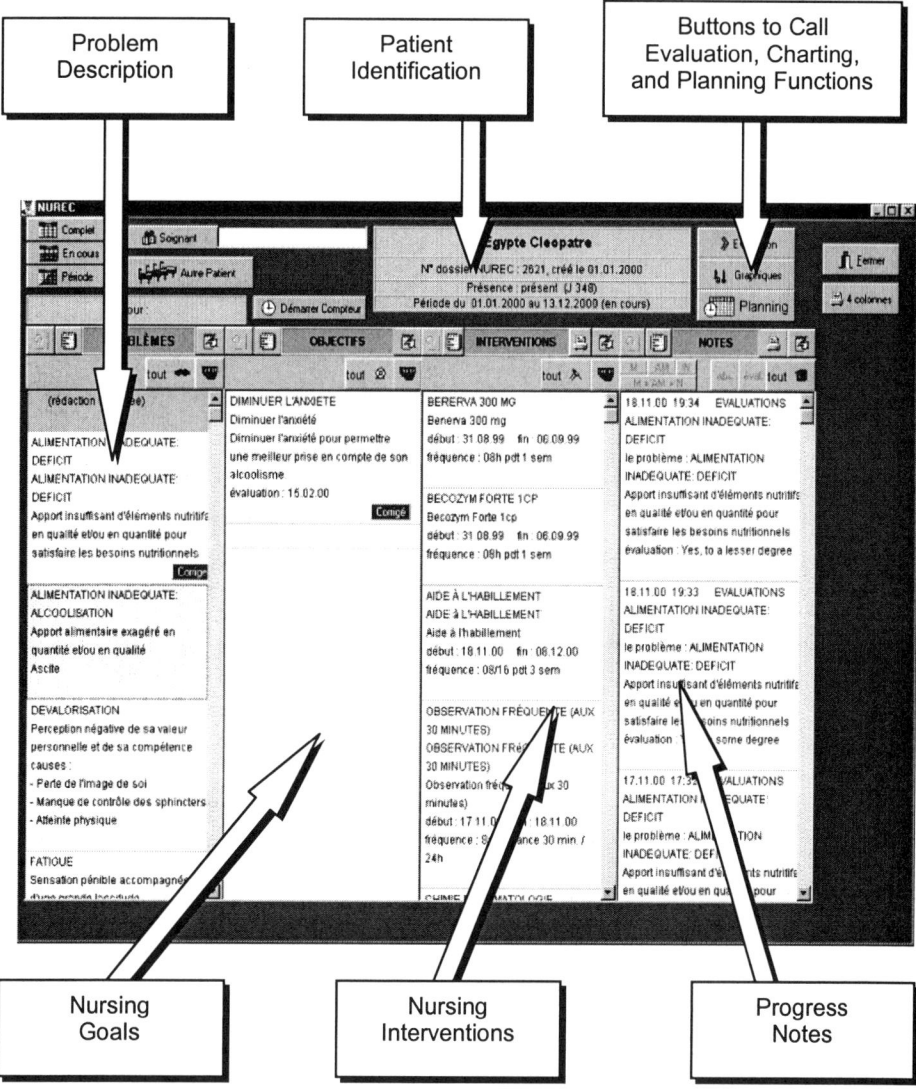

Figure 10. Problem Editing and Intervention Scheduling

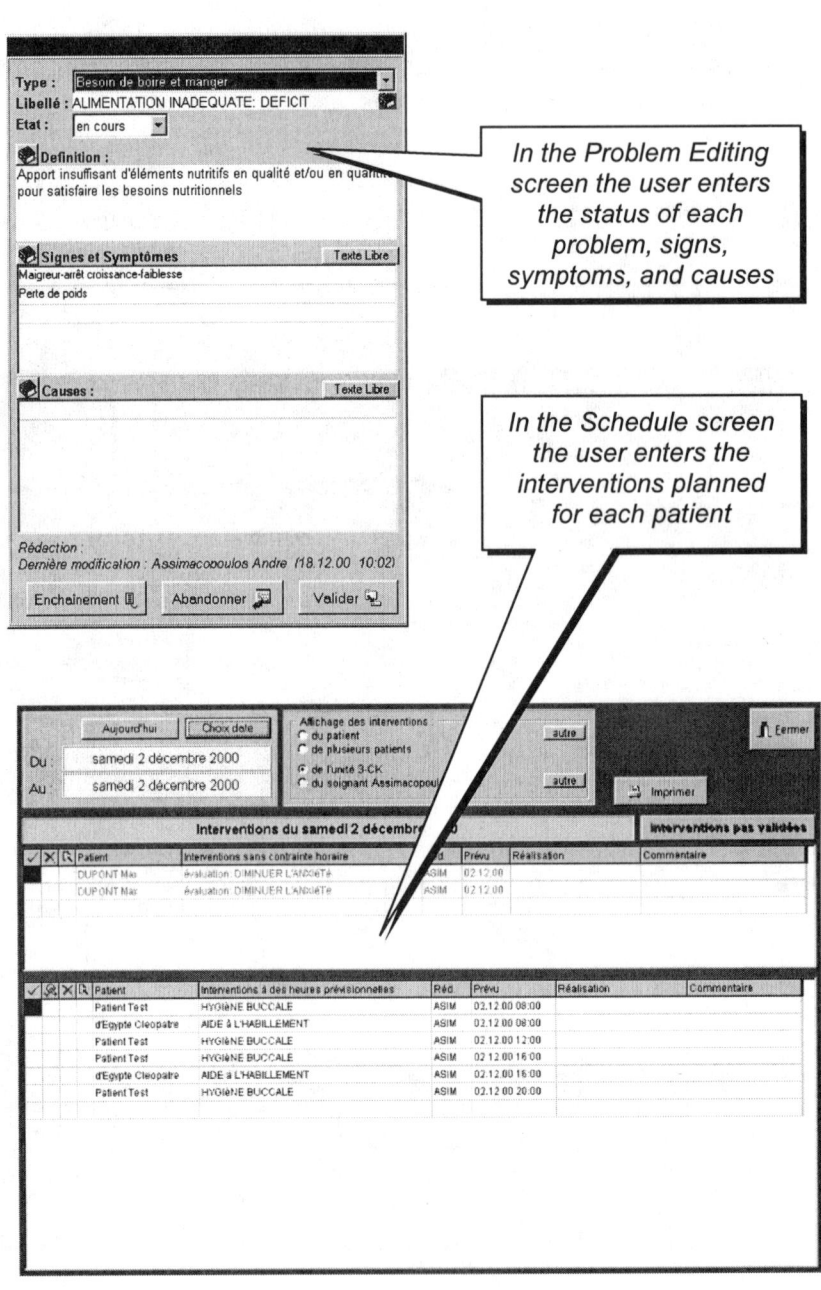

Figure 11. Degree of Importance of Problem and Vital Signs

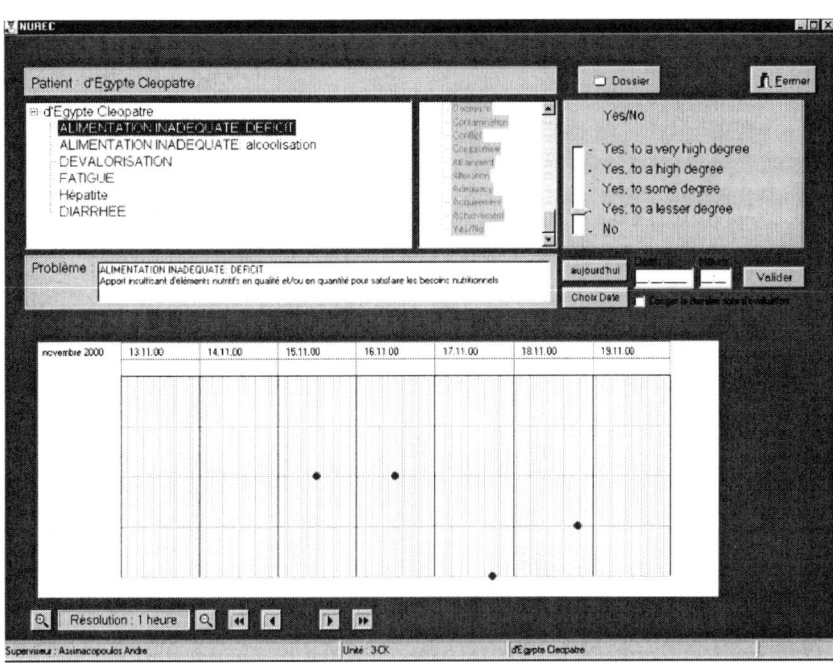

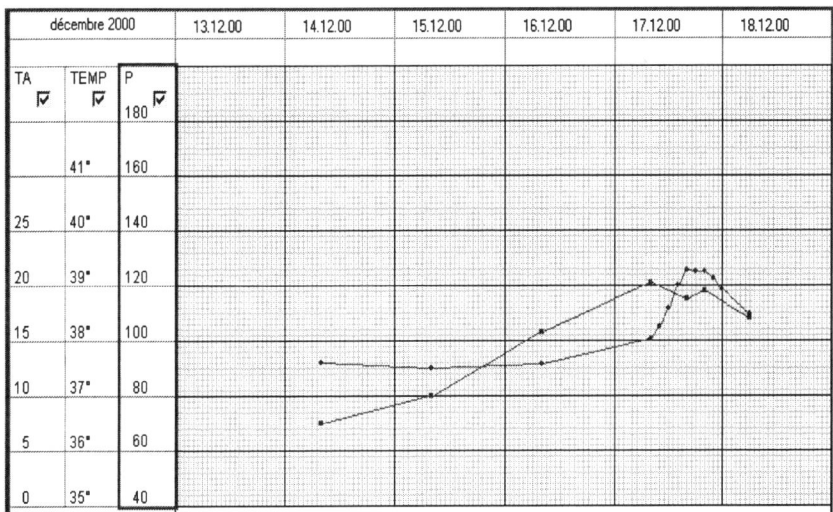

7.   Education and Research in Nursing Informatics

Nurses constitute the largest group of health professionals in any health system. However, to this day the group has not been well served regarding nursing informatics education. The American Nurses Association (ANA) officially recognized this discipline as a nursing specialty in 1992 when it defined the scope of practice for Nursing Informatics (Saba and McCormick, 1996; ANA, 1995a; ANA, 1998b). It is a sobering finding that after nearly twenty years of effort by nursing informatics enthusiasts in the United Kingdom only a small proportion of the nursing and midwifery professions have become active in applying nursing informatics to their field of practice (Barnett, 1995).

7.1.   Educating Nurses in Informatics

Nursing informatics education may be viewed from three requirement perspectives: nurse academics needing computers, information, and telecommunication technologies to support teaching and research; nurses requiring those technologies to support their daily practice; and finally nursing informatics education required to prepare nurse informaticians. Each of these requirements demands its own and distinctive educational program. The mission for all nurse educators is to enable nurses to use health, medical, and nursing information together with telematics (informatics and telecommunication technologies) to enhance global health, health service delivery, and health system effectiveness.

According to Barnett (1999) it is likely to be well into the next decade before all nurses have had the opportunity to learn more about informatics. Education in informatics is primarily being provided by Nursing Computer/Informatics groups through short courses, seminars, and focused conferences. Few countries offer Nursing Informatics as a postgraduate specialist program. In the United States, a list of the educational programs that offer Nursing Informatics can be found on the American Medical Informatics Association Web site (www.amia.org). Examples in Latin America and the Caribbean are the programs of the Nursing Informatics Group at the Federal University of São Paulo (NIEn/UNIFESP), Brazil, and the Diploma Program in Health Information at the Barbados Community College, in Barbados, West Indies.

7.2.   A Competence-based Educational Framework

Gonczi et al. (1993) defined professional competence as "having the attributes necessary for job performance to the appropriate standards". Competency-based education is specific to the learner's requirements to do a given job, and is currently used by many healthcare facilities to measure competence in the nursing role.

Competence is viewed as a simultaneous integration of the knowledge, skills, and attitudes required for the performance in a designated role or setting (Fearon, 1998). Defining successful professional performance requires an analysis of the role and tasks performed. To assist this decision-making process, performance criteria need to be developed that are clearly defined. Professional competencies should be established in order to evaluate and refine the education of the users. These competencies should be built into the existing framework of the educational process. In this way, the competency-based training enables the learners to easily assess their areas of strength and weakness.

Competencies required for the various staff positions will vary, as each of these groups is expected to perform different roles and functions; this will be reflected in the differing competency requirements delineated for each increasing level of responsibility. This requires the educators to emphasize a learner's ability to demonstrate the proficiencies that are of central importance to their own specific task or activity. Competence-building activities will include sensitization programs, training of nursing staff, and continuous education opportunities.

Changes in the workplace command corresponding educational processes to facilitate those changes. The educational process in current facilities may need to be expanded to include the new areas discussed in this document. Training programs must prepare students for the nurse's growing role in providing care, and nurses need to integrate computers into their daily routine. The required curricula will equip nurses at all levels and in all roles to become more sophisticated in using computer technology to support clinical decision making and delivery of care. (Zielstorff et al., 1993; Rodrigues and Malik, 1993). The current generation of nurses will benefit from the increasing use of computer technology in the traditional nursing schools, but nurses already working in healthcare settings will have to gain this knowledge through continuing education channels or staff development (Rodrigues, 1984). Those involved in staff development face the challenge of educating staff of various levels of computer and information literacy.

Acquisition of knowledge and desired skills by health personnel is necessary for the full participation of end-users in the development process. They are the best insurance for a successful implementation of a functional nursing information system. The existence of information system support staff at all healthcare delivery levels is critical to the success of the program (Rodrigues, 1983; Rodrigues, 1986; Rodrigues, 1988).

The following strategic guidelines are recommended in preparing nurses for the use of data standards and computer-based applications:

- A structured human resource development program will be developed to increase awareness, assess training needs, and build capacity and competencies for designing and implementing data standards;

- Implementation planning should ensure that staff involved in all levels of project implementation and operation will receive appropriate training, both theoretical and practical, in data standards, health information systems, and the management of information functions in organizations;

7.3. Educational Tools

A great variety of new educational technologies are available that can profitably be used to develop courseware materials and in the training and education the nursing staff. Examples are: multimedia or computer-based technologies that allow an integration of traditional forms of communication to provide seamless access or interaction by the users (Hannah et al., 1999); computer-assisted instruction (CAI); interactive video (IAV); and CD-ROM instruction. These tools ideally reside in a special learning resource center that provides the resources for education. This allows flexible and self-administered education and training for the various staff or students.

Other computer-based tools focus on literature databases such as MEDLINE (Medlars Online), CINAHL (Cumulative Index Nursing and Allied Health Literature), and other databases with nursing-related literature. The Internet offers several online protocols that can support the transmission of data, including: electronic mail (E-mail), file transfer protocol (FTP), Telnet and the World Wide Web (WWW). The WWW allows nurses to access resources from anywhere around the world. All of these can be used to enhance nursing education and healthcare (Saba and McCormick, 2001).

> *Computer-based tools are most useful in knowledge and information transfer processes, providing feedback to students about the efficiency of the learning process, and in permitting access to a vast warehouse of electronic databases. This enables students to solve problems and apply their learning (Hannah et al., 1994).*

Distance learning can be utilized to train large number of nurses in different geographic locations and work settings. Tools for distance education include Web-based courses (synchronous and asynchronous), teleconferencing (individual or group) or combinations of both.

Computerized clinical simulation has many potential uses in education and as a testing tool for licensure examination. Interactive software permits the realistic assessment and management of client needs through free-text entry of requests for nursing activities, each of which can elicit a response – the efficiency and accuracy of the particular application, however, is dependent on the careful structuring of a comprehensive nursing activity database (Bersky and Krawczak, 1995).

7.4. Curriculum Development

Practicing nurses should have a minimum of computer-based education established in their curriculum. In addition to the use of computers to teach nursing content, the use of the computer as an information tool in the clinical area should be integrated into the daily aspects of nursing care, clinical laboratory systems, pharmacology information, and physician orders. In order to educate current nursing staff about the use of computers, training strategies must take into account the nurses' level of training and experience.

> *Nursing Informatics education needs to address four critical issues: (a) Foremost is the diversity of possible content due to the many combinations of foundation disciplines. When combined and given a nursing information focus, these make up (b) an increasingly complex discipline. In addition, there is (c) a shortage of suitable educators, and they would all acknowledge the difficulty of adding any new material to existing nursing curricula. Finally, (d) students entering Nursing Informatics programs possess variable levels of computing knowledge and skills, ranging from those who have never switched on a computer to those who are able to write programs.*

Nurses with little or no previous experience in data standards and computer technology should receive basic training in the use of computer- supported nursing information systems, computer applications in nursing practice, in the selection, production, and evaluation of software, and in managing computer-supported information systems.

Nurses with basic training and more experience in data standards should participate in programs that focus on the institutionalization of the nursing information system. Content of this program could include topics such as current status and quality of the solution utilized, analysis and utilization of standards data in the improvement of nursing practice, and approaches in evaluating the impact of the nursing information system.

For student nurses, a formal education in Nursing Informatics such as a specific Nursing Informatics Specialization Course or a Master's or Doctoral Degree should be offered.

7.5.   Research in Informatics

The establishment of and active research program in nursing informatics assures the development and evaluation of nursing informatics solutions to the challenges of contemporary patient care (Barreira y Castro and Almeida, 1985; Brennan et. al, 1998).

Priorities for research include projects that address the following topics: nursing information requirement analysis and systems specification, systems functionalities and modeling, formalization of nursing vocabularies, design and management of databases for nursing information, telecommunications and interactive communications technologies applications, direct-care patient applications, patient use of information technology in the care environment, and evaluation of feasibility, appropriateness, and impact of nursing information systems. To establish and maintain their leadership, researchers should emphasize the investigation of potential applications of emerging technologies to nursing practice.

The Sigma Theta Tau International (STTI) Honor Society of Nursing supports one of the most important registries of nursing research. The Society is dedicated to improving the health of people worldwide through increasing the scientific base of nursing practice. To achieve this goal, STTI is committed to furthering the use of nursing research in health care delivery as well as in public policy. It sustains, supports, and interprets nursing development and provides vision for the future of the discipline and health care through its network of worldwide community of nurse scholars. More than a quarter million nurse scholars have been inducted into STTI. With 120,000 active members, it is the second largest nursing organization in the world. Members are active in more than 90 countries and territories.

The Registry of Nursing Research is an electronic research resource that is maintained by Sigma Theta Tau International (STTI), Honor Society of Nursing. It contains information and abstracts from over 13,000 studies. Research findings are indexed by variable or phenomenon of study and can be searched by keywords (RNR, 2001).

8.   References

– ANA (American Nurses Association). Standards of Practice in Nursing Informatics. Washington, DC, 1995a.

– ANA (American Nurses Association). An Emerging Framework: Data System Advances for Clinical Nursing Practice. Washington, DC: ANA, 1995b.

– ANA (American Nurses Association). Nursing Information and Data Set Evaluation Center (NIDSEC): Standards and Scoring Guidelines. NIDSEC Committee (Zielstorff R, Delaney C, Marek K, Kneedler J, Marr P, Averrill C, Milholand K and ANA staff). Washington, DC, 1997.

– ANA (American Nurses Association). Standards of Clinical Nursing Practice. 2nd ed. Washington, DC, 1998a.

– ANA (American Nurses Association). Scope of Practice for Nursing Informatics. Washington, DC, 1998b.

– Angerami EL, Carvalho EC. [Nursing process: reflections on the terminology used]. (Article in Portuguese). Rev Esc Enfermagem USP 1987; 21:29-33.

– Alselmi ML, Carvalho EC, Angerami EL. [Nursing history: theory and practice of its understanding and use]. (Article in Portuguese). Rev Esc Enfermagem USP 1988; 22(2):181-188.

– Bakken S, Cashen MS, Mendonca E, O'Brien A, Zieniewicz J. Representing nursing activities within a concept-based terminologic system: evaluation of a type definition. J Am Med Inform Assoc 2000; 7:81-90.

– Ball MJ, Snelbecker GE. Overcoming resistance to tele-communications innovations in medicine and continuing medical education. Computers in Hospitals 1982; 3(4):40-45.

– Ball MJ. Integration of systems for patient care. In: Hovenga EJS, Hannah KJ, McCormick KA, Ronald JS (eds.). Nursing Informatics '91: Proceedings of the Fourth International Conference on Nursing Use of Computers and Information Science, Melbourne, Australia, April 14-17, 1991. Lecture Notes in Medical Informatics Volume 42: Springer-Verlag, Berlin, Heidelberg: pages 110-114; 1991a.

– Ball MJ, Douglas JV, O'Desky RI, Albright JW. Healthcare Information Management Systems: A Practical Guide. Springer-Verlag, New York; 1991b.

– Barnett DE. Informing the nursing professions about IT. In: Greenes RA, Peterson HE, Protti DJ (eds.). Proceedings of the Eighth World Congress on Medical Informatics, Vancouver, Canada: IMIA and Healthcare Computing & Communications, Canada Inc, Edmonton; 1995.

– Barnett DE. Tomorrow is only a vision. ITIN 1999; 11(1):8-11.

– Barreira y Castro I, Almeida MC. [Nursing research as instrument for change in practice and manpower training]. (Article in Spanish). Educ Méd Salud 1985; 19(3):313-136.

– Bersky AK, Krawczak J. Building a nursing activity database for processing free-text entry during computerized clinical simulation testing. Comput Nurs 1995; 13(5):236-243.

– Beya, S. Standardized nursing vocabularies and the perioperative nursing data set: making clinical practice count. CIN Plus 2000; 3(2):5-6.

– Brennan PF, Zielstorff RD, Ozbolt JG, Strombom I. Setting a national research agenda in nursing informatics. Medinfo 1998; 9 Part 2:1188-1191.

– Buckovich SA. Privacy, confidentiality, and security. In: Saba VK, McCormick KA (eds.). Essentials of Computers for Nurses: Informatics for the New Millennium. 3rd edition. McGraw-Hill, New York; 2001.

– Button P, Androwich I, Hibben L, Kern V, Madden G, Marek K, Westra B, Zingo C. Challenges and issues related to implementation of nursing vocabularies in computer-based systems. J Am Med Inform Assoc 1998; 5(4):332-334.

– Campbell J, Carpenter P, Sneiderman C, Cohn S, Chute C, Warren J. Phase II evaluation of clinical coding schemes: Completeness, taxonomy, mapping, definitions, and clarity. J Am Med Inform Assoc 1997; 4(3):238-251.

– Campbell KE, Cohn SP, Chute CG, Shortliffe EH, Rennels G. Scalable methodologies for distributed development of logic-based convergent medical terminology. Meth Inform Med 1998; 37:426-439.

– Carpenito LJ. [Nursing Diagnosis; Practice Application], (Article in Portuguese). 6th edition., Porto Alegre, Artes Médicas; 1997.

– CEN (Comité Europeen de Normalisation). ENV 12264: Medical Informatics - Categorical Structures of Systems of Concepts. Model for Representation of Semantics. Brussels, Belgium: CEN - European Committee for Standardization; 1997.

– CEN (Comité Europeen de Normalisation). PrENV 14032: Health Informatics – System of Concepts to Support Nursing. Revised Final Draft. CEN/TC 251/N00-083. CEN/TC 251 Secretariat: SIS-HSS (Swedish Healthcare Standards Institution): Stockholm; 2000.

– Ceusters W. Harmonisation and formalisation of nursing terminology: A three dimensional approach. In: Mortensen RA (ed.) ICNP and Telematic Applications for Nurses in Europe: The Telenurse Experience. Amsterdam: IOS Press, 1999;164-173.

– Chute CG, Cohn SP, Campbell KE, Oliver DE, Campbell JR. The content coverage of clinical classifications. J Am Med Inform Assoc 1996; 3:224-233.

– Chute CG, Cohn SP, Campbell JR. A framework for comprehensive terminology systems in the United States: Development guidelines, criteria for selection, and public policy implications. ANSI Healthcare Informatics Standards Board Vocabulary Working Group and the Computer-based Patient Records Institute Working Group on Codes and Structures. J Am Med Inform Assoc 1998; 5:503-510.

– Chute CG. Terminology services as software components: An architecture and preliminary efforts. In: Chute CG (ed.) Proceedings of IMIA Working Group 6 Medical Concept Representation and Natural Language Processing. Phoenix: International Medical Informatics Association, 1999; 62-69.

– Cimino JJ. Desiderata for controlled medical vocabularies in the twenty-first century. Meth Inform Med 1998; 37:394-403.

– Cimino JJ. Terminology tools: State of the art and practical lessons. In: Chute CG (ed.). Proceedings of IMIA Working Group 6 Medical Concept Representation and Natural Language Processing. Phoenix: International Medical Informatics Association 1999; 218-228.

99

– Clark J, Lang NM. Nursing's next advance: An international classification for nursing practice. Int Nurs Rev 1992; 39:109-112.

– Clark J, Delaney C. Conceptualization and Feasibility of an International Nursing Minimum Data Set (i-NMDS). In: Saba VK, Carr R, Sermeus W, Rocha P (eds.). One Step Beyond: The Evolution of Technology and Nursing. Proceedings of the 7th International Congress on Nursing Informatics; 2000.

– Clark J, Craft-Rosenberg, M, Delaney C. An international methodology to describe clinical nursing phenomena: a team approach. Int J Nurs Studies 2000; 37:541-553.

– Collier IC, McCash KE, Bartram JM. Writing Nursing Diagnoses – a Critical Thinking Approach. Mosby, St. Louis: Missouri; 1996.

– Council of Europe. Directive 95/46/EC of the European Parliament and of the Council of 24 October 1995 on the Protection of Individuals with Regard to the Processing of Personal Data and on the Free Movement of such Data. 1995. Available from: http://www.privacy.org/pi/intl_orgs/ec/eudp.html

– Craft-Rosenberg M, Delaney C, Denehy J. Nursing Diagnosis Extension Classification (NDEC): history, methods, completed work, and future directions. In: Rantz M, LeMone P (eds.). Classification of Nursing Diagnoses: Proceedings of the Thirteenth Conference NANDA. Glendale, CA: CINAHL Information Systems; 2000.

– Cruz IC. [Nursing diagnosis and its application: review of the literature]. (Article in Portuguese). Rev Esc Enfermagem USP 1990a; 24(1):149-162.

– Cruz IC. [Pilot study on the implementation of the nursing process in a post-anesthesia recovery unit]. (Article in Portuguese). Rev Esc Enfermagem USP 1990b; 24(3):345-358.

– Cruz IC, Cruz D. [Human response patterns: a proposal for the translation to Portuguese of the terms of the nursing diagnosis taxonomy I]. (Article in Portuguese). Rev Esc Enfermagem USP 1991; 25(1):17-20.

– Cruz DAL. [Nursing diagnosis in teaching and research]. (Article in Portuguese). Rev Esc Enfermagem USP 1992; 26(3):427-434.

- Dalri, MC. [Diagnostic profile of burn patients according to the conceptual model of Horta and the NANDA revised taxonomy]. (Article in Portuguese). Dissertation for Master's Degree. Escola de Enfermagem de Ribeirão Preto. Universidade de São Paulo; 1993.

- Delaney C, Huber D. A Nursing Management Minimum Data Set (NMMDS): a report of an invitational conference. Chicago, IL: American Organization of Nurse Executives; 1996.

- Delaney C, Reed D, Clarke M. Describing patient problems and nursing treatment patterns using Nursing Minimum Data Sets (NMDS & NMMDS) and UHDDS repositories. In: Overhage JM (ed.). AMIA 2000 Converging Information, Technology and Health Care; 2000: 176-179).

- Dias CB. [Observation in nursing: the need for a concept]. (Article in Portuguese). Master's Degree Dissertation. Escola de Enfermagem de Ribeirão Preto. Universidade de São Paulo; 1990.

- Doenges ME, Moorhouse MF, Burley JT. Application of Nursing Process and Nursing Diagnoses. F.A. Davis Company, USA, 1992.

- Ehnfors M. Testing the ICNP in Sweden and other Nordic countries. In: Mortensen RA (ed.). ICNP and Telematic Applications for Nurses in Europe: The Telenurse Experience. Amsterdam: IOS Press; 1999:221-229.

- Ehnfors M, Hardiker N, Hoy D, Nielsen G, Therkelsen L, Rossi Mori A. CEN/TC 251 Short Strategic Study. Systems of concepts for nursing: a strategy for progress. Final Report: European Standardisation Committee (CEN); 1999.

- Eng TR, Gustafson DH. (eds.) Wired for Health and Well-Being - The Emergence of Interactive Health Communication. US Department of Health and Human Services: Science Panel on Interactive Communication and Health; Office of Public Health and Science. Washington,DC: US Printing Office; 1999.

- European Union. European Commission Group on Ethics in Science and New Technologies. Ethical Issues of Healthcare in the Information Society. Report #13, Wagner I (Rapporteur);1999 July 30. Available from: http://europa.eu.int/comm/secretariat_general/sgc/ethics/en/opinion13.pdf.

- Evora, YD. [Nursing and Informatics: Present Trends and Future Perspectives]. (Article in Portuguese). Dissertation for Doctoral Degree. Escola de Enfermagem de Ribeirão Preto, Universidade de São Paulo; 1993.

- Fearon M. Assessment and measurement of competence in practice. Nursing Standard 1998;12(22):43-47.

- Friedlander MR. [The nursing process yesterday, today, and tomorrow]. (Article in Portuguese). Rev Esc Enfermagem USP 1981; 15(2):129-134.

- Gassert CA. A focus on implementing nursing vocabularies. J Am Med Inform Assoc 1998; 5(4):390.

- Gir E, Carvalho EC, Ferraz AE. [Function and role: study of terminology]. (Article in Portuguese). Rev Gauch Enfermagem 1990; 11(1):11-17.

- Goethe B. [Proposal of a protocol for the care of the newborn infant with hyaline membrane disease respiratory insufficiency at the Hospital Regional Simón Bolívar in Bogotá]. (Article in Spanish). Document of the Hospital Regional Simón Bolívar, Bogotá. Colombia: July 1989.

- Gonczi A, Hager P, Athanasou J. The Development of Competency-Based Assessment Strategies for the Professions. Research Paper No. 8 Department of Employment, Education and Training. AGPS Canberra; 1993.

- Goodman KW. Ethics, Computing and Medicine: Informatics and the Transformation of Health Care. Cambridge University Press; 1998.

- Grenade P. Telemedicine: a look at the legal issues confronting a new delivery system. Kilpatrick and Cody Medical Law Update. Winter 1996.

- Grobe SJ. The Nursing Intervention Lexicon and Taxonomy: Implications for representing nursing care data in automated records. Hol Nurs Prac 1996; 11(1):48-63.

- Guirao i Goris JA, Cuesta A, Benavent A. [Nursing diagnosis: keys for its development]. (Article in Spanish). Rev Enferm 1999; 22(7-8):554-558.

- Gutierrez BA, López AL, Cruz DAL, Souza TT. [Agreement between terms of the nursing problem list and the International Classification of Nursing Problems, alpha version]. (Article in Portuguese). Rev Med Hosp Univ 1999; 9(1):37-44.

- Hannah KJ, Ball MJ, Edwards JA. Introduction to Nursing Informatics. Springer-Verlag, New York; 1994.

– Hardiker NR, Hoy D, Casey A. Standards for nursing terminology. J Am Med Inform Assoc 2000; 7(6):523-528.

– Henry SB, Holzemer WL, Reilly CA, Campbell KE. Terms used by nurses to describe patient problems: Can SNOMED III represent nursing concepts in the patient record? J Am Med Inform Assoc 1994; 1:61-74.

– Henry SB, Mead CN. Nursing classification systems: necessary but not sufficient for representing "what nurses do" for inclusion in computer-based patient record systems. J Am Med Inform Assoc 1997; 4(3):222-232.

– Henry SB, Elfrink V, McNeil B, Warren J. The ICNP's relevance in the US. Int Nurs Rev 1998a; 45:153-158.

– Henry SB, Warren J, Lange L, Button P. A review of the major nursing vocabularies and the extent to which they meet the characteristics required for implementation in computer-based systems. J Am Med Inform Assoc 1998b; 5(4):321-328.

– Herrero T, Cabrero AI, Burgos MR, Garcia M, Fernandez AI. [Quality control in nursing records]. (Article in Spanish). Enferm Intensiva 1998; 9(1):10-15.

– Hodge JG Jr, Gostin LO, Jacobson PD. Legal issues concerning electronic health information: privacy, quality, and liability. JAMA 1999; 282(15):1466-1471.

– Huber D, Delaney C. Nursing management data for nursing information systems. In: Series on Nursing Administration (SONA), Information Systems Innovations: New Visions, New Ventures 1998; Volume 10:15-29.

– Huff SM, Carter JS. A characterization of terminology models, clinical templates, message models, and other kinds of clinical information models. In: Chute CG (ed.). Proceedings of International Medical Informatics Association Working Group 6 Conference on Natural Language and Medical Concept Representation. Phoenix: International Medical Informatics Association; 1999:74-82.

– ICN (International Council of Nursing). Nursing's next advance: an international classification for nursing practice (ICNP) - a working paper, Genebra; 1993.

– ICN (International Council of Nursing). International classification for nursing practice (ICNP) - alpha version, Genebra; 1996.

– ICN (International Council of Nurses). ICNP Update. Geneva, Switzerland: International Council of Nurses; 1999.

– IITF (Information Infrastructure Task Force). Privacy and the NII: Safeguarding Telecommunications-Related Personal Information. Report of the Information Infrastructure Task Force (IITF). Washington, DC: US Department of Commerce, National Telecommunications and Information Agency; 1995.

– Impicciatore P, Pandolfini C, Casella N, Bonati M. Reliability of health information for the public on the World Wide Web: systematic survey of advice on managing fever in children at home. BMJ. 1997;314(7098):1875-1879.

– IHC (Internet Healthcare Coalition). Minutes of the Internet Healthcare Coalition e-Health Ethics Summit. Internet Healthcare Coalition e-Health Ethics Summit; 2000 Jan 31-Feb 2; Washington(DC). 2000. Available from: http://www.ihealthcoalition.org/ethics/ehcode.html

– ISECS (Instituto Superior de Acreditación para el Desarrollo de la Enfermería y otras Ciencias de la Salud). [Project Nursing Standards - prNE IG 14. Interventions Defined for Diagnostic Related Groups 14] (Document in Spanish). ISECS: Madrid; January 2001.

– ISO (International Standards Organization). Proposed Scope of Work: Integration of a reference terminology model for nursing. Geneva, Switzerland: International Standards Organization; 1999.

– Iyer PW, Camp NH. Nursing Documentation: a Nursing Process Approach. 3rd edition, Mosby, St. Louis, Missouri; 1999.

– Jesus CAC. [A conceptual framework for the nursing care of hematologic patients]. (Article in Portuguese). Dissertation for Master's Degree. Escola de Enfermagem de Ribeirão Preto. Universidade de São Paulo; 1992.

– Jesus CAC. [Historial evolution of nursing diagnosis and its applicability in care planning]. (Article in Portuguese). Rev Saúde Dist Fed 1995; 6(1-2):37-40.

– Johnson M, Maas M (eds.). Nursing Outcomes Classification (NOC). Mosby, St. Louis, Missouri; 1997.

– Johnson M, Maas M, Moorhead S (eds.). Nursing Outcomes Classification (NOC). 2nd ed. St. Louis, Missouri; 2000.

– Johnson M, Bulechek G, Dochterman-MacCloskey J, Maas M, Moorhead S. Nursing Diagnoses, Interventions, and Outcomes: NANDA, NIC, and NOC Linkages. Mosby, St. Louis, Missouri; 2001.

– Lang NM, Brooten D. The quality of health care: from traditional to innovative practice. In: Nursing in the Americas. Pan American Health Organization, PAHO/WHO, Washington, DC, 1999. ISBN 92 75 11571 0.

– Lewin K. Quasi-stationary social equilibria and the problem of permanent change. In: Bennis WG, Benne KD, Chin R. (eds.) The Planning of Change . Holt, Reinhart, and Winston, New York; pages 235-238;1969.

– Luis MV, Scochi CGS, Atzingen RH. [Reflexions on the insertion of informatics in the nursing profession]. (Article in Portuguese). Rev Gauch Enfermagem 1992; 13(1):37-40.

– Mandil SH. Health informatics should influence, and be influenced by its key components: the example of nursing practice. In: Hovenga EJS, Hannah KJ, McCormick KA, Ronald JS (eds.). Nursing Informatics '91: Proceedings of the Fourth International Conference on Nursing Use of Computers and Information Science, Melbourne, Australia, April 14-17, 1991. Lecture Notes in Medical Informatics Volume 42: Springer-Verlag, Berlin, Heidelberg: pages 21-28; 1991.

– Manfredi M, Souza AM. [Nursing education in Latin America]. (Article in Spanish). Educ Méd Salud 1986; 20(4):473-484.

– Manfredi, M. [The development of nursing in Latin America: a strategic view]. (Article in Spanish). Rev Lat Am Enfermagem 1993; 1(1):23-35.

– Martin KS, Scheet NJ. The Omaha System: Applications for Community Health Nursing. Saunders, Philadelphia; 1992.

– Martin KS, Scheet, NJ. The Omaha System: Applications for Community Health Nursing. 2nd edition. Saunders, Philadelphia; 1995.

– Martin KS, Norris J. The Omaha System: a model for describing practice. Holist Nurs Pract 1996; 11(1):75-83.

– Mayes R. Data Standards. In: Saba VK, McCormick KA. Essentials of Computers for Nurses: Informatics for the New Millennium. 3rd edition. McGraw-Hill, New York; 2000.

– McCloskey JC & Bulechek GM. Nursing Intervention Classification. 1st edition. Mosby, St. Louis, Missouri; 1992.

– McCloskey JC, Bulechek GM. Nursing Interventions Classification. 2nd edition. Mosby, St. Louis, Missouri ; 1996.

– McCloskey JC, Bulechek GM. Nursing Interventions Classification. 3rd edition. Mosby, St. Louis, Missouri ; 2000.

– McCormick K. A unified nursing language system. In: Ball, MJ, Hannah KJ, Gerdin Jelger U, Peterson H (eds.). Nursing Informatics: Where Caring and Technology Meet. Springer-Verlag, New York; pages 168-178; 1988.

– McCormick K. The urgency of establishing international uniformity of data. In: Hovenga EJS, Hannah KJ, McCormick KA, Ronald JS (eds.). Nursing Informatics '91: Proceedings of the Fourth International Conference on Nursing Use of Computers and Information Science, Melbourne, Australia, April 14-17, 1991. Lecture Notes in Medical Informatics Volume 42: Springer-Verlag, Berlin, Heidelberg: pages 77-81; 1991.

– McCormick K, Lang N, Zielstorff R, Milholland DK, Saba VK, Jacox A. Toward standard classification schemes for nursing language: Recommendations of the American Nurses Association Steering Committee on Databases to Support Nursing Practice. J Am Med Inform Assoc 1994; 1:421-427.

– McHugh ML. Computer system. In: Saba VK, McCormick KA (eds.). Essentials of Computers for Nurses: Informatics for the New Millennium. 3rd edition. McGraw-Hill, New York; 2001.

– Moen A, Henry SB, Warren JJ. Representing nursing judgments in electronic health records. J Adv Nurs 1999; 30(4):990-997.

– Mortensen RA, Nielsen GH. International Classification of Nursing Practice (version 0.2). Geneva, Switzerland: International Council of Nursing; 1996.

– Mortensen RA. ICNP in Europe towards the year 2000 TelenurseID. In: Mortensen RA (ed.). ICNP and Telematic Applications for Nurses in Europe: The Telenurse Experience. IOS Press, Amsterdam; 1999:3-6.

– NANDA (North American Nursing Diagnoses Association). Nursing Diagnoses: Definitions and Classifications 1995-1996. North American Nursing Diagnosis Association, Philadelphia, PA; 1993.

– NANDA (North American Nursing Diagnoses Association). Nursing Diagnoses: Definitions and Classification 1999-2000. North American Nursing Diagnosis Association, Philadelphia, PA; 1999.

– Nielsen GH. Mortensen RA. The architecture for an international classification for nursing practice (ICNP). International Nursing Review 1996; 43(6):175-82.

– Nielsen GH. PART I. Telenurse introduction to α-ICNP. In: The International Classification for Nursing Practice (ICNP) with TELENURSE Introduction. Alpha Version. Danish Institute for Health and Nursing Research, Copenhagen; 1996.

– Nielsen GH. The architecture of ICNP. In: Mortensen RA. (Ed.) ICNP in Europe. Telenurse. Studies in Health Technology and Informatics. IOS Press, Amsterdam; pages13-29; 1997.

– Nielsen GH. Mortensen RA. The architecture for an international classification for nursing practice (ICNP). Time for Outcomes. Part I. International Nursing Review 1997a; 44(7):182-89.

– Nielsen GH. Mortensen RA. The architecture for an international classification for nursing practice (ICNP). Time for Outcomes. Part II. International Nursing Review 1997b; 45(7):27-31.

– Nielsen GH. The Telenurse Introduction to β-ICNP. Danish Institute for Health and Nursing Research, Copenhagen; 1999.

– Nielsen GH. Towards the beta ICNP: Processes and Products. In: Mortensen RA (Ed.) ICNP and Telematic Applications for Nurses in Europe. The Telenurse Experience. Studies in Health Technology and Informatics. IOS Press, Amsterdam; pages 13-31; 1999a.

– Nielsen GH, Mortensen RA. ICNP time for outcomes: Continuous quality development. In: Mortensen RA (ed.). ICNP and Telematic Applications for Nurses in Europe: The Telenurse Experience. IOS Press, ; Amsterdam; 1999b:79-102.

– Nobrega MM, Coler MS. [Mapping of Horta's basic human needs theory to NANDA classification of nursing diagnoses]. (Article in Portuguese). CCS 1994; 13(3):86-92.

107

– PAHO (Pan American Health Organization). [Investigation on nursing labor force in six countries]. (Article in Spanish). Educ Méd Salud 1988; 22(1):64-90.

– PAHO (Pan American Health Organization). Information Systems and Information Technology in Health: Challenges and Solutions for Latin America and the Caribbean. Health Services Information Systems Program. PAHO/WHO, Washington, DC; April 1998. ISBN 92 75 12246 6.

– PAHO (Pan American Health Organization). Setting Up Healthcare Services Information Systems: A Guide for Requirement Analysis, Application Specification, and Procurement. Essential Drugs and Technology Program, Division of Health Systems and Services Development. PAHO/WHO, Washington, DC; 1999a. ISBN 92 75 12266 0.

– PAHO (Pan American Health Organization). [Nursing in the Region of the Americas]. (Article in Spanish). Serie Organización y Gestión de Sistemas y Servicios de Salud, Volume 16. División de Desarrollo de Sistemas y Servicios de Salud. PAHO/WHO, Washington, DC; 1999b.

– PAHO (Pan American Health Organization). Framework for a Comparative Analysis of the Changes in Nursing Practice, Regulation and Education in the Context of Health Care Reform. Series Organization and Management of Health Systems and Services. Division of Health Systems and Services Development, Volume 20. PAHO/WHO, Washington, DC; 2000a.

– PAHO (Pan American Health Organization). Nursing for Equity, Access, Quality, and Sustainability in the Health Services. Division of Health Systems and Services Development, Washington, DC; 2000b (in press).

– Pascal A, Frecon-Valentin E. [Nursing care. The evolution of nursing classification]. (Article in French). Soins 1998; (627):10-13.

– Perez VL, Nóbrega MM, Farias JN, Coler MS. [Nursing diagnosis: a challenge to nursing in the 90's]. (Article in Portuguese). Rev Bras Enfermagem 1990; 43(1-4):14-18.

– RNR (Registry of Nursing Research). Sigma Theta Tau International; 2001. Available online at: http://www.nursingsociety.org/

– Robazzi ML, Moriya TM, Ferraz AE, Carvalho EC, Bachion MM. [The application of NANDA Taxonomy I in nursing diagnoses in a workers environment]. (Article in Portuguese). Rev Baiana Enfermagem 1995; 8(1-2):5-20.

– Rodrigo MT. [Nursing diagnosis]. (Article in Spanish). Rev Enferm 1997; 20(222):26-31.

– Rodrigues MA. [Continuing education in public health nursing]. (Article in Portuguese). Rev Esc Enfermagem USP 1984; 18(2):129-140.

– Rodrigues RJ. The human element in systems development. In: De Talens AFP et al. (eds.). Health Informatics and Developing Countries: Experiences and Viewpoints. Proceedings of the IFIP-IMIA World Congress on Medical Informatics and Developing Countries, North-Holland: pages139-147; 1983.

– Rodrigues RJ. Introducing microcomputers to health professionals in a large public hospital environment. In: Salamon R, Blum R, Jorgensen M (eds.). Proceedings of the Fifth Conference on Medical Informatics (MEDINFO 86), IFIP-IMIA, North-Holland: pages 380-384; 1986.

– Rodrigues RJ. [The educational component in the development of human resources for health informatics]. (Article in Portuguese). Rev Bras Informatica Saúde 1988; 1(5):10-11.

– Rodrigues RJ, Goihman S. [Information system for the management of local health systems]. (Article in Portuguese). Bol Of Sanit Panam 1990; 109(5-6):488-501.

– Rodrigues RJ, Malik AM (eds.). Preparing Health Care Managers for a Changing World - What is our Role?. Proceedings of the International Seminar in Health Administration, University of Chile. W.K.Kellogg Foundation and INSORA. Santiago; Oct 1-7, 1993. ISBN 9 567424 01 2.

– Rodrigues RJ, Israel K. Conceptual Framework and Guidelines for the Establishment of District-Based Information Systems. PAHO/WHO Office of Caribbeam Program Coordination, Bridgetown, Barbados; 1995. (Publication PAHO/CPC/3.1/95.1). ISBN 976-8083-75-1.

– Rodrigues RJ, Oxman G, Israel K, Priale, R. [Conceptual framework for the deployment of local helath information systems]. (Article in Spanish). HSS/SILOS/UNI Volumen 8, PAHO/WHO; 1995.

– Rodrigues RJ, Crawford C, Koss S, McDonald M. Telecommunications in Health and Healthcare for Latin America and the Caribbean. Series Health Services Information Systems/ HSP, No. 1, PAHO/WHO; 1997

– Rodrigues RJ. Ethical and legal issues in interactive health communications: a call for international cooperation (Editorial). J Med Internet Research 2000a; 2 (1). Available online at: http://www.jmir.org/2000/1/index.htm.

– Rodrigues RJ. Telemedicine and the transformation of healthcare practice in the information age. In: Speakers' Book of the International Telecommunication Union (ITU) Telecom Americas 2000; Telecom Development Symposium, Session TDS.2; Rio de Janeiro, April 10-15, 2000b, pages 91-105.

– Rodrigues RJ. Information systems and evidence-based practice. In: Proceedings of the Eighth National and Sixth International Conference on Information Technology in Community Health (ITCH2000), University of Victoria, Victoria, BC, Canada, August 23-27, 2000c. ISBN 1 55058 216 X.

– Rodrigues RJ. Information systems: the key to evidence-based health practice. Bull World Health Org 2000d; 78 (11):1344-1351.

– Roos PN, Roos LL, Mossey J, Havens B. Using administrative data to predict important health outcomes: entry to hospital, nursing home, and death. In: White K, Frenk J, Ordoñez C, Paganini JM, Starfield B (eds.). Health Services Research: An Anthology. Pan American Health Organization, Washington, DC; 1992. (Scientific Publication No. 534).

– Rossi LA, Dalri MCB. [Nursing process in a burn service: analysis and reformulation proposal utilizing Horta and NANDA nursing diagnosis classification]. (Article in Portuguese). Rev Esc Enfermagem USP 1993; 27(3):328-354.

– Ryan P, Delaney C. The Nursing Minimum Data Set: research findings and future directions. In: Annual Review of Nursing Research, Springer Publishing New York, NY, Volume 13: pages 169-194; 1995.

– Saba VK. Home health care classification system. In: Mortensen R (ed.). Creating a European Platform - Proceedings of the First European Conference on Nursing Diagnoses. Copenhagen: pages 302-308; 1995a.

– Saba VK. Home Health Care Classifications (HHCCs): Nursing Diagnoses and Nursing Interventions. In: ANA Database Committee. Nursing Data Systems: The Emerging Framework. Washington, DC: ANA: pages 55-60; 1995b.

– Saba VK, McCormick KA . Essentials of Computers for Nurses. McGraw-Hill, New York; 1996.

- Saba VK. Nursing information technology: classification and management. (Unpublished paper). Georgetown University School of Nursing, Washington, DC; 1999.

- Saba VK, McCormick KA (eds.). Essentials of Computers for Nurses: Informatics for the New Millennium. 3rd edition. McGraw-Hill, New York; 2001.

- Schanz SJ (ed.) 1999 Compendium of Telemedicine Laws - Selected Statute Excerpts and Article Citations Relating to Telemedicine. Legamed Inc., Raleigh, NC;1999. ISBN 0 965 7439 2 6.

- Scochi CGS, Santos BRL, Evora YDM. [Informatics in nursing practice: a new challenge to the nurse] (Article in Portuguese). Rev Gauch Enfermagem 1991; 12(2):19-22.

- Scochi CGS, Rodríguez R, Luis M, Evora YD, Moala FA. [The teaching of informatics in nursing]. (Article in Spanish). Horiz Enferm 1993; 4(1):42-49.

- Silberg WM, Lundberg GD, Musacchio RA. Assessing, controlling, and assuring the quality of medical information on the Internet: caveant lector et viewor – let the reader and viewer beware. JAMA. 1997; 277(15):1244-5.

- Simões N. [Professional metalanguage: the elaboration of a technical and scientific vocabulary for nursing]. (Article in Portuguese). Dissertation for Doctoral Degree. Escola de Enfermagem de Ribeirão Preto. Universidade de São Paulo; 1988.

- Simões C. [Outline of a conceptual structure for nursing]. (Article in Portuguese). Rev Paul Enfermagem 1992; 11(2):59-63.

- Soberón G, Herrera F, Nájera RM. [Primary care nursing in Mexico]. (Article in Spanish). Educ Méd Salud 1984; 18(1):34-45.

- Sosa-ludicissa M, Oliveri N, Gamboa CA, Roberts J. (eds.). Internet, Telematics and Health. Studies in Health Technology and Informatics: Volume 36. PAHO/WHO and IMIA: IOS Press; 1997. ISBN 90 5199 289 0.

- Soto PE, Ramos E, Alonso C, Navea M, Refusta L, Echevería E. [Course: informatics as iupport to nursing management]. (Article in Spanish). In: Congreso Chileno de Sociedades Científicas de Enfermería. Ponencias y resúmenes. 1992; 70-71.

- Stanberry BA. Legal and ethical issues in european telemedicine. European Telemedicine. 1998/99; 20-25.

111

– UNESCO (United Nations Educational, Scientific and Cultural Organization). Report of the Experts Meeting on Cyberspace Law, Sept 29-30 1998; Monte-Carlo, Principality of Monaco. Document CII/USP/ECY/99/01; 1999.

– Vasquez MA, Bueno M, Casals JL, Garcia JM. [Nursing diagnosis of risks. Analysis of cost-effectiveness]. (Article in Spanish). Rev Enferm 1998; 21(237):26-32.

– Villalobos NA. [Implementation of the nursing process at the operative level]. (Article in Spanish). Rev Lat Am Enfermagem 1999; 7(1):67-73.

– Werley HH, Lang NM (eds.). Identification of the Nursing Minimum Data Set. Springer, New York; 1995.

– WHO (World Health Organization). Informatics and Telematics in Health: Present and Potential Uses. Geneva; 1988. ISBN 92 4 156117 3.

– WHO (World Health Organization). A Health Telematics Policy in Support of WHO's Health-for-All Strategy for Global Health Development. Report of the WHO Group Consultation on Health Telematics; 1997 Dec 11-16. Publication WHO/DGO/98.1; 1998.

– WHO (World Health Organization). Design and Implementation of Health Information Systems. Lippeveld T, Sauerborn R, Bodart C (eds.). World Health Organization, Geneva: 2000. ISBN 92 4 1561998.

– Wright MG. [A common language for nurses: a persistent dilemma]. (Article in Spanish). Rev Lat Am Enfermagem 1995; 3(2):107-129.

– Yoshioca MR, Barbosa MA, Narchi NZ; Cruz IC, Bezerra AL, Imanichi RM. [International classification of nursing activities: a sample of the Brazilian reality]. (Article in Portuguese). Rev Bras Enfermagem 1993; 46(3-4):258-265.

– Yoshioca MR, Barbosa MA, Rocha MT, Rossato LM, Regina VL, Farias FA, Rodrigues AM. [Development of databases to support nursing activities]. (Article in Portuguese). Rev Esc Enfermagem USP 1994; 28(1):27-40.

– Zanetti ML, Marziale MH, Robazzi ML. [Horta's model and NANDA's taxonomy and problem solving strategy in nursing care]. (Article in Portuguese). Rev Gauch Enfermagem 1994; 15(1-2):76-84.

–   Zaragoza A. [The nursing process. Perspectives of teachers and alumnae]. (Article in Spanish). Rev Enferm 1999; 22(9):582-590.

–   Zielstorff RD, Hudgings CI, Grobe SJ. Next Generation Nursing Information Systems: Essential Characteristics for Practice. Washington, DC: American Nurses Association; 1993.

APPENDIX 1.

Summarizing Tables of Systems and Organizations

Tables prepared and included in this document thanks to Dr. Suzanne Bakken

Table 1. Types of Systems of Concepts for Nursing

TYPE OF SYSTEM	SEMANTIC CATEGORIES	RELATIONSHIPS AMONG CONCEPTS	TERMS	PRIMARY PURPOSE	EXAMPLE
Interface Terminology	Typically implicit	Typically implicit	Present	Ease of data entry	Omaha System
Administrative Terminology (Classification System)	Explicit	Explicit, generic	Present	Statistical classification	Nursing Interventions Classification
Reference (Formal) Terminology	Explicit	Explicit, generic, partitive, associative	Present	Non-ambiguous concept definition	SNOMED RT
Categorical Structure	Explicit	Explicit, generic, partitive, associative	Absent	Describe semantic categories for development, maintenance, and application of terminological systems	Categorical structures proposed in Short Strategic Study
Terminology Model	Explicit	Explicit, associative	Absent	Terminology organization and management	Attributes of fully-specified Clinical LOINC name
Reference Information Model	Explicit	Explicit, generic, associative	Absent	Information system development / standards for information sharing	"Loose Cannon" Model for Nursing Interventions
Semantic Archetype	Explicit	Explicit, associative	Absent	Incorporates aspects of use (e.g., record structure) in organization of concepts	Generic semantic archetype for nursing assessment

Table 2. Organizations Focused on Standards Development or Facilitation

ORGANIZATION	A	B	C	D	E	F	G
Accredited Standards Committee (ASC) X12 and X12N	✓	✓					
American College of Radiology/National Electrical Manufacturers Association (ACR/NEMA)	✓	✓					
American Dental Association (ADA)	✓						
American Medical Association (AMA)	✓						
American Nurses Association (ANA)	✓			✓			
American National Standards Institute Health Care Informatics Standards Board (ANSI-HISB)	✓	✓	✓				✓
American Society for Testing and Materials (ASTM)	✓	✓	✓				✓
College of American Pathologists/SNOMED	✓						
Computer-based Patient Record Institute (CPRI)	✓						✓
European Standardization Committee (CEN)	✓	✓	✓	✓	✓	✓	✓
Health Care Financing Administration (HCFA)	✓						✓
Health Level 7 (HL7)	✓	✓	✓		✓	✓	✓
Institute of Electrical and Electronic Engineers (IEEE)		✓					
International Council of Nurses	✓						
International Standards Organization (ISO)	✓	✓	✓	✓	✓	✓	✓

A = Standardized Healthcare Terminologies
B = Decision Support
C = Messaging
D = Minimum Data Sets
E = Categorical Structures and Terminology Models
F = Health Record Architecture
G = Privacy, Confidentiality, and Security

Table 3. Terminologies for Representing Concepts of Relevance to the Nursing Domain

TERMINOLOGY	PROBLEMS/ DIAGNOSES	INTERVEN- TIONS	GOALS AND OUTCOMES	CRITICAL ANALYSES
Current Procedural Terminology (1)		✓		Campbell (2), Griffith (6), Henry (10)
Home Health Care Classification[1] (28)	✓	✓	✓	Henry (11), Holzemer (13)
International Classification of Nursing Practice (25)	✓	✓	✓	Henry (12), Marin (19), Ehnfors (5)
National Health Service (NHS) Clinical Terms (Read Codes) (3)	✓	✓	✓	Campbell (2), Humphreys (14)
North American Nursing Diagnosis Association Taxonomy I[1] (26)	✓			Campbell (2), Chute (4), Henry (11), Moen (24)
Nursing Intervention Lexicon and Taxonomy[1] (7)		✓		
Nursing Interventions Classification[1] (21, 22)		✓		Hardiker (8), Henry (11)
Nursing Outcomes Classification[1] (15, 16)			✓	
Omaha System[1] (20)	✓	✓	✓	Henry (11)
Patient Care Data Set[1] (27)	✓	✓		McDaniel (23)
Perioperative Nursing Data[1] (17)	✓	✓	✓	
SNOMED International, SNOMED RT[1] (29)	✓	✓	✓	Campbell (2), Chute (4), Henry (9), Lange (18), Humphreys (14)

[1] ANA recognition indicates that a request for evaluation and documentation regarding the reliability, validity, ability to be implemented in computer-based systems, and utility for nursing practice of a terminology has been submitted to the ANA and that the terminology meets the ANA criteria in these areas (McCormick K, Lang N, Zielstorff R, Milholland DK, Saba VK, Jacox A. Toward standard classification schemes for nursing language: Recommendations of the American Nurses Association Steering Committee on Databases to Support Nursing Practice. J Am Med Inform Assoc 1994; 1:421-427.)

Numbers in parentheses point to references listed in the following page.

Reference Citations for Table 3.

1. American Medical Association. Physician's Current Procedural Terminology. Chicago; 1993.

2. Campbell J, Carpenter P, Sneiderman C, Cohn S, Chute C, Warren J. Phase II evaluation of clinical coding schemes: Completeness, taxonomy, mapping, definitions, and clarity. J Am Med Inform Assoc 1997; 4:238-251.

3. Casey A. The UK clinical terms projects and quality improvement. In: Henry SB, Holzemer WL, Tallberg M, Grobe S (eds.). Informatics: The Infrastructure for Quality Assessment and Improvement in Nursing. UC Nursing Press, San Francisco; 1995: 21-23.

4. Chute CG, Cohn SP, Campbell KE, Oliver DE, Campbell JR. The content coverage of clinical classifications. J Am Med Inform Assoc 1996; 3:224-233.

5. Ehnfors M. Testing the ICNP in Sweden and other Nordic countries. In: Mortensen RA, (ed.) ICNP and Telematic Applications for Nurses in Europe: The Telenurse Experience. IOS Press, Amsterdam; 1999; 221-229.

6. Griffith HM, Robinson KR. Current Procedural Terminology (CPT) coded services provided by nurse specialists. Image 1993; 25:178-186.

7. Grobe SJ. The Nursing Intervention Lexicon and Taxonomy: Implications for representing nursing care data in automated records. Hol Nurs Prac 1996; 11(1):48-63.

8. Hardiker N, Kirby J. A compositional approach to nursing terminology. In: Gerdin U, Tallberg M, Wainwright P, eds. Nursing Informatics: The Impact of Nursing Knowledge on Health Care Informatics. Stockholm: IOS Press, 1997; 4-7.

9. Henry SB, Holzemer WL, Reilly CA, Campbell KE. Terms used by nurses to describe patient problems: Can SNOMED III represent nursing concepts in the patient record? J Am Med Inform Assoc 1994; 1:61-74.

10. Henry SB, Holzemer WL, Randell C, Hsieh S-F, Miller TJ. Comparison of Nursing Interventions Classification and Current Procedural Terminology codes for categorizing nursing activities. Image 1997; 29:133-138.

11. Henry SB, Warren J, Lange L, Button P. A review of the major nursing vocabularies and the extent to which they meet the characteristics required for implementation in computer-based systems. J Am Med Inform Assoc 1998; 5:321-328.

12. Henry SB, Elfrink V, McNeil B, Warren J. The ICNP's relevance in the US. Int Nurs Rev 1998; 45:153-158.

13. Holzemer WL, Henry SB, Dawson C, Sousa K, Bain C, Hsieh S-F. An evaluation of the utility of the Home Health Care Classification for categorizing patient problems and nursing interventions from the hospital setting. In: Gerdin U, Tallberg M, Wainwright P, eds. Nursing Informatics: The Impact of Nursing Knowledge on Health Care Informatics. Stockholm: IOS Press,1997; 21-26.

14. Humphreys BL, McCray AT, Cheh ML. Evaluating the coverage of controlled health data terminologies: Report on the results of the NLM/AHCPR Large Scale Vocabulary Test. J Am Med Inform Assoc 1997; 4:484-500.

15. Johnson M, Maas M, eds. Nursing Outcomes Classification (NOC). Mosby, St. Louis; 1997.

16. Johnson M, Maas M, Moorhead S, eds. Nursing Outcomes Classification (NOC). 2nd ed. Mosby, St. Louis; 2000.

17. Kleinbeck SVM. In search of perioperative nursing data elements. AORN J 1996; 63:926-931.

18. Lange L. Representation of everyday clinical nursing language in UMLS and SNOMED. In: Cimino JJ, (ed.) Proceedings of the AMIA Fall Symposium. Hanley & Belfus Inc., Philadelphia; 1996;140-144.

19. Marin HF. Translating and testing ICNP in Brazil. In: Mortensen RA (ed.) ICNP and Telelmatic Applications for Nurses in Europe: The Telenurse Experience. IOS Press, Amsterdam; 1999; 254-257.

20. Martin KS, Scheet NJ. The Omaha System: Applications for Community Health Nursing. Saunders, Philadelphia; 1992.

21. McCloskey JC, Bulechek GM. Nursing Interventions Classification. 2nd ed. Mosby, St. Louis; 1996.

22. McCloskey JC, Bulechek GM. Nursing Interventions Classification. 3rd ed. Mosby, St. Louis; 2000.

119

23. McDaniel AM. Developing and testing a prototype patient care database. Comput Nurs 1997;15:129-136.

24. Moen A, Warren JJ, Henry SB. Representing nursing judgments in electronic health records. J Adv Nurs 1999; 30:990-997.

25. Mortensen RA, Nielsen GH. International Classification of Nursing Practice (version 0.2). Geneva, Switzerland: International Council of Nursing; 1996.

26. NANDA. Nursing Diagnoses: Definitions and Classification 1999-2000. Philadelphia: North American Nursing Diagnoses Association, 1999.

27. Ozbolt JG. From minimum data to maximum impact: Using clinical data to strengthen patient care. Adv Prac Nurs Q 1996; 1(4):62-69.

28. Saba VK, Zuckerman AE. A new home health classification method. Caring Magazine 1992; 11(9):27-34.

29. Spackman KA, Campbell KE, Cote RA. SNOMED RT: A Reference Terminology for health care. In: Masys D (ed.) Proceedings of the 1997 AMIA Annual Fall Symposium. Hanley & Belfus Inc., Philadelphia; 1997: 640-644.

APPENDIX 2.

Nursing Management Minimum Data Set (NMMDS)

Delaney C, Huber, D. A Nursing Management Minimum Data Set (NMMDS): A Report of an Invitational Conference. Chicago, IL: American Organization of Nurse Executives; 1996.

Delaney C, Reed D, Clarke M. Describing Patient Problems and Nursing Treatment Patterns using Nursing Minimum Data Sets (NMDS and NMMDS) and UHDDS repositories. In Overhage JM (ed.). AMIA 2000 Converging Information, Technology, and Health Care, pages 176-179; 2000.

NMMDS – Environment

Variable	Definition
1. Type of nursing delivery unit or service	Unique name and identifier of a center of excellence, service program, cluster by level of care, service/product line, service/area where majority of patient/client care is delivered; the first level of data aggregation beyond the patient/client care provider.
2. Patient/client population	Characteristics, including specialty, development, interaction, and population foci of patient/client population served by nursing delivery unit or service
3. Volume of nursing delivery unit or service	Amount of provided and available service to an individual, family, group, or community/population by a nursing delivery unit or service.
4. Nursing delivery unit or service accreditation.	Recognition of nursing delivery or unit service by relevant accrediting body.
5. Decisional participation	Extent to which decision-making power is distributed throughout the organization.
6. Unit or service complexity	Perceived extent of environmental factors impacting the nursing delivery unit or service.
7. Patient/client accessibility	Time and distance required for nursing or patient/client care support personnel of the nursing delivery unit/service to reach the point of care.
8. Method of care delivery	Predominant method of organizing the delivery and accountability of patient/client care by the nursing delivery unit or service.
9. Complexity of clinical decision making	Degree of routineness, uniformity, predictability, and knowledge involved in delivering nursing care/service; consideration is given to frequency of activities and whether required procedures are well understood by providers.

NMMDS – Nurse Resources

Variable	Definition
10. Manager demographic profile	Demographics of the leadership of the nursing delivery unit or service; demographics of the person by whatever title, designated as the nurse manager with 24 hour administrative accountability for a nursing delivery unit or service; includes span of control and number of people the manager is responsible for directing, even if not under span of control in budget.
11. Nursing staff and client care support personnel	Number of staff available to provide direct and indirect services to a nursing delivery unit or service population.
12. Nursing care staff demographic profile	Education and experience profile of nursing care staff.
13. Nursing care staff satisfaction	Percentage of care personnel by classification who report positive or negative affect toward their job.

NMMDS – Financial Resources

Variable	Definition
14. Payer type	Type, effort, and revenue for each payer for care delivered by nursing unit or service, total nursing, and total healthcare facility.
15. Reimbursement	Distribution formula/payment for services within nursing delivery unit or service.
16. Nursing delivery unit or service budget	Organization total annual itemized budget for a nursing delivery unit or service compared to the nursing delivery unit or service total annual itemized actual allocation.
17. Expenses	Direct and indirect cost per nursing delivery unit/service per year.

APPENDIX 3.

Health and Communications Standards

1.   Healthcare Standards and Classification Systems: a Brief Review

It is a great challenge to build a clinical vocabulary that standardizes the medical nomenclature for use in clinical practice, fulfills all of the requirements of indexed retrieval, and promotes fast communication. Cimino et al. (1994) point out that a clinical vocabulary, to be effective, needs to be complete, unambiguous, precise, and non-redundant. Furthermore, clinical vocabularies need to be represented in such a way that synonyms and relationships can be explicitly represented, and they must use data structures that allow multi-axial classification. However, clinical vocabularies must be simple to understand, easy to encode, and intuitive to apply.

Main obstacles to the creation and use of a general-purpose controlled clinical vocabulary are:

- Clinical language is constantly evolving (a moving target);

- Inadequacy of expression of relationship among terms, and term modifiers;

- Regional and international differences;

- Inadequacy of software tools.

Standards developing organizations and committees have developed several classification systems. Most of them are being used to code, document, classify, and label care that has been given to the patient/client inside and outside of a hospital. The ones most widely used are briefly described.

International Statistical Classification of Diseases and Related Health Problems, Tenth Revision (ICD-10)

The ICD-10, published by the World Health Organization (WHO), is the latest revision of a system of categories to which diseases and related health conditions are assigned according to established criteria. The classification is the most-used standard for classifying mortality and morbidity conditions and is utilized in the compilation of statistical reports and comparison of health status among different health institutions, regions, and countries. This classification is accepted worldwide and comprises not only diagnostic labels but also a nomenclature structure. The International Classification of Diseases has been revised and updated periodically.

Current Procedural Terminology (CPT codes)

The CPT codes are developed and maintained by the American Medical Association (AMA), being widely used in the United States of America for reimbursement and review purposes. Nurses routinely use many of the CPT codes. In a recent study, seven nursing groups (family care, midwifery, school, orthopedics, oncology, rehabilitation, and critical care) indicated that they use 493 codes to document as well as to be reimbursed for the services they provide. Similar coding schemes have been developed and used by healthcare systems in Latin American. The main purpose for those codes of medical procedures has been the payment for services provided by physicians.

The Systematized Nomenclature of Human and Veterinary Medicine (SNOMED and SNOMED International

SNOMED is a structured nomenclature and classification of terminology used in human and veterinary medicine. The code structure is developed and maintained by the College of American Pathologists (CAP) and is widely accepted for describing pathological test results. It has a multi-axial coding structure that gives it greater clinical specificity than the ICD and CPT codes, and has considerable value for clinical purposes. SNOMED is being used by an increasing number of healthcare providers in several countries.

SNOMED International contains eleven modules. Each module comprises an independent taxonomy that includes topography; morphology; function; living organisms; chemical, drugs and biological products; physical agents; occupations; social context; disease/diagnosis; procedures; and general linkage/modifiers. It is interesting to point out that SNOMED is adding nursing terms to their nomenclature.

Unified Medical Language System (UMLS)

The United States National Library of Medicine (NLM) maintains this system. It contains a metathesaurus that links biomedical terminology, semantics, and formats of the major clinical coding and reference systems. It associates medical terms (ICD, CPT, SNOMED and others) to the NLM Medical Index Subject Headings (MeSH codes) and to each other. The UMLS also contains a specialist lexicon that can be identified as a Metathesaurus of Terms and Concepts from various vocabularies of the different databases; a Semantic Network of the relationships among the broad categories to which the concepts of the metathesaurus are assigned; and an Information Sources Map of machine-readable biomedical databases. Together, those elements should represent all codes, vocabularies, terms, and concepts and will become the foundation for an emerging medical informatics infrastructure. Currently, at least four nursing classification schemes recommended by the American Nurses Association (ANA) Database Steering Committee are included on the UMLS.

There are many other vocabularies, code sets, and classification systems being developed and implemented around the world, e.g., the Logical Observation Identifier Names and Codes (LOINC), the International Medical Terminology, Read Codes, Diagnostic and Statistical Manual of Mental Disorders, etc. For an extensive review of classification standards refer to PAHO's publication *"Setting Up Healthcare Services Information Systems: A Guide for Requirement Analysis, Application Specification, and Procurement"*. Essential Drugs and Technology Program, Division of Health Systems and Services Development. PAHO/WHO, Washington, D.C., July 1999, ISBN 92 75 12266 0.

2.   Communications Standards

Data Communication standards address, primarily, the format of messages exchanged between computer systems and the coding and classification schemes used within the message. In order to achieve data compatibility between systems, it is necessary to have prior agreement on the syntax of the messages that will be exchanged. The receiving system must be able to parse the incoming message into discrete data elements which reflect what the sending system wishes to communicate.

There are different standards for different kinds of message depending upon the subject matter and method of communication. Four broad classes of message format standards have emerged in the healthcare sector: medical device communications; digital imaging communications; administrative data exchange; and clinical data exchange. Organizations, private groups, or government agencies are developing communications standards. A list of the most important follows:

International Standards Organization (ISO)

Oversees the development of standards internationally. It is a worldwide federation of national standards organizations. The purpose is to promote the development of standardization and related activities internationally.

American National Standards Institute (ANSI)

The Institute serves as the coordinator of voluntary standards activities in the United States and is the agency that approves standards as American National Standards.

Comité Europeen de Normalisation (CEN)

CEN is a European standard organization with 16 Technical committees. Two of them are specifically involved in healthcare area: TC 251 (Medical Informatics) and TC 224 WG12 (patient data cards).

Institute of Electrical and Electronic Engineers (IEEE)

The IEEE has developed a series of standards known collectively as P1073 Medical Information Bus (MIB) which support real time, continuous, and comprehensive capture and communication of data from bedside medical devices such as those found in Intensive Care Units, Operating Rooms, and Emergency Departments. These data include physiological parameter measurements and devices settings.

Digital Imaging Communication in Medicine Standards Committee (DICOM)

The National Electrical Manufactures Association (NEMA), the American College of Radiologists (ACR), and others formed DICOM with the objective of developing a generic digital format and transfer protocol for biomedical images and image-related information. The specification can be used on any type of computer system and supports transfer over the Internet. The DICOM standard is the dominant international data interchange message format in biomedical imaging. It is also incorporated into the European MEDICOM (Medical Image Communication) standard and Japanese "second common" standard for medical communications over networks.

American Society for Testing and Materials (ASTM)

The ASTM E31.12 Computer-based Patient Records Subcommittee is responsible for content and structure of the Computer Patient Record and Computer Patient Record Systems. This committee has been involved in developing standards for electronic patient records, defining the organization of the information, the meaning of the terms, and the logical structure of the patient record.

Accredited Standards Committee (ASC) X-12N Committee

The committee is responsible for the development of a range of Electronic Data Interchange (EDI) standards to facilitate electronic business transactions. In the healthcare arena, the X12N standard was proposed for adoption as national standards for administrative transactions, enrollment and eligibility in health plans insurance. Due to the uniqueness of health insurance practices from country to country, these standards are primarily used in the United States.

Health Level 7 (HL7)

Focus on standards for transmitting and communicating clinical data within and across institutions. It has established several technical committees and special-interest groups, which meet periodically to develop data standards. Major areas covered by the standard include medical orders; clinical observations; test results; admission, transfer, and discharge; and charge and billing information.

APPENDIX 4.

Further Reading – a Complementary List of References on Nursing Informatics, Standards, Terminologies, and Related Subjects

– Alternate Billing Concepts. Las Cruces, New Mexico: Alternate Link LLC; 1998.

– Alvarez M, Figueroa M, Flores M, Moya C, Muñoz LA. [Project CIPE in Chile 1997-1999]. (Article in Spanish). Colegio de Enfermeras de Chile; 1999.

– Assimacopoulos A, Balahoczky M, Junod B, Kruezsely A, Borgazzi A. Using the electronic nursing record NUREC-CH for workload management: Results and integration perspectives. In: Mortensen RA (ed.). ICNP and Telematic Applications for Nurses in Europe: The Telenurse Experience. IOS Press, Amsterdam; 1999; 111-118.

– Bakken S. Integrating nursing concepts into SNOMED RT/SNOMED CT. Presentation to the SNOMED Users Group. Washington, DC; 1999.

– Ball MJ, Hannah, KJ. Using Computers in Nursing. Reston, VA: Reston Publishers; 1984.

– Braithwaite W. HIPAA and the Administration Simplification Law. MD Computing 1999; 16:13-16.

– Brown PJB, Price C. Semantic-based concept differential retrieval & equivalence detection in Clinical Terms Version 3 (Read Codes). In: Lorenzi N (ed.) Proceedings of AMIA '99 Annual Symposium. Hanley & Belfus Inc.: Philadelphia; 1999; 27-31.

– Button P, Mead CN, Warren JJ, Androwich I, Bakken S. The Loose Cannon Information Model of Nursing Interventions. In: Saba VK (ed.) Proceedings of NI 2000; (in press).

– Camus, L. [Information system to support clinical evidence in nursing]. (Article in Spanish). Pontificia Universidad Católica de Chile, Escuela de Enfermería. Unpublished document; 2000

– Carter B. Development of an educational model for computer instruction. In: Hovenga EJS, Hannah KJ, McCormick KA, Ronald JS (eds.). Nursing Informatics '91: Proceedings of the Fourth International Conference on Nursing Use of Computers and Information Science, Melbourne, Australia, April 14-17, 1991. Lecture Notes in Medical Informatics Volume 42: Springer-Verlag, Berlin, Heidelberg: 1991; 465-469.

– Casey A. The UK Clinical Terms Projects and quality improvement. In: Henry SB, Holzemer WL, Tallberg M, Grobe S (eds.). Informatics: The Infrastructure for Quality Assessment and Improvement in Nursing. San Francisco: UC Nursing Press, 1995; 21-23.

– Cimino JJ, Hripcsak G, Johnson SB, Clayton PD. Designing an introspective, multi-purpose, controlled medical vocabulary. In: Kingsland III LC (ed.). Proceedings of the 13th Symposium on Computer Applications in Medical Care. Washington, DC: IEEE Computer Society Press, 1989; 513-518.

– Clark J. Note from the president. ACENDIO Newsletter 1999; 5:1-2.

– College of American Pathologists. SNOMED International: the Systemized Nomenclature of Human and Veterinary Medicine. Northfield, IL; 1993.

– Corn M. Funding for nursing vocabularies [editorial]. J Am Med Inform Assoc 1998; 5:391-392.

– Ehnfors M, Thorell-Ekstrand I, Ehrenberg A. Towards basic nursing information in patient records. Vard i Norden 1991; 3/4:12-31.

– Fawcett-Henesy A. Surveillance of peoples need for nursing care using electronic sampling – A WHO perspective. In: Mortensen RA (Ed.) ICNP and Telematic Applications for Nurses in Europe. The Telenurse Experience. Studies in Health Technology and Informatics. Amsterdam. IOS Press; 1999: 199-203.

– Forsythe D. An anthropologist's viewpoint: Observations and commentary regarding implementation of nursing vocabularies in computer-based systems. J Am Med Inform Assoc 1998; 5(4):329-331.

– Gassert C. Validating a model for defining nursing information systems requirements. In: Hovenga EJS, Hannah KJ, McCormick KA, Ronald JS (eds.). Nursing Informatics '91: Proceedings of the Fourth International Conference on Nursing Use of Computers and Information Science, Melbourne, Australia, April 14-17, 1991. Lecture Notes in Medical Informatics Volume 42: Springer-Verlag, Berlin, Heidelberg: 1991; 215-219.

– Gassert C. A focus on implementing nursing vocabularies [editorial]. J Am Med Inform Assoc 1998; 5(4):390.

– Gaston C. The politics of nursing information systems and resource allocation. In: Hovenga EJS, Hannah KJ, McCormick KA, Ronald JS (eds.). Nursing Informatics '91: Proceedings of the Fourth International Conference on Nursing Use of Computers and Information Science, Melbourne, Australia, April 14-17, 1991. Lecture Notes in Medical Informatics Volume 42: Springer-Verlag, Berlin, Heidelberg: 1991; 3-13.

– Griffith HM, Robinson KR. Survey of the degree to which critical care nurses are performing Current Procedural Terminology-coded services. Am J Crit Care 1992; 1:91-98.

- Griffith HG, Robinson KR. Current Procedural Terminology (CPT) coded services provided by nurse specialists. Image 1993; 25(3):178-186.

- Hardiker N, Kirby J. A compositional approach to nursing terminology. In: Gerdin U, Tallberg M, Wainwright P (eds.). Nursing Informatics: The Impact of Nursing Knowledge on Health Care Informatics. Stockholm: IOS Press; 1997: 4-7.

- Hardiker NR, Rector AL. Modeling nursing terminology using the GRAIL representation language. J Am Med Inform Assoc 1998; 5(1):120-128.

- Helena M. Nursing data in the hospital integrated information system SONHO. In: Mortensen RA (ed.). ICNP and Telematic Applications for Nurses in Europe: The Telenurse Experience. Amsterdam: IOS Press; 1999:137-143.

- Heller BR, Braun RF, Moray LR, Gassert CA, Romano CA. Evaluation of a prototype graduate level program of study in nursing informatics. In: Hovenga EJS, Hannah KJ, McCormick KA, Ronald JS (eds.). Nursing Informatics '91: Proceedings of the Fourth International Conference on Nursing Use of Computers and Information Science, Melbourne, Australia, April 14-17, 1991. Lecture Notes in Medical Informatics Volume 42: Springer-Verlag, Berlin, Heidelberg: 1991; 653-659.

- Henry SB. Clinical decision making in critical care: the relationship among computer simulation performance, cognitive examination, and sel-assessment of expertise. In: Hovenga EJS, Hannah KJ, McCormick KA, Ronald JS (eds.). Nursing Informatics '91: Proceedings of the Fourth International Conference on Nursing Use of Computers and Information Science, Melbourne, Australia, April 14-17, 1991. Lecture Notes in Medical Informatics Volume 42: Springer-Verlag, Berlin, Heidelberg: 1991; 226-230.

- Henry SB, Holzemer WL, Randell C, Hsieh S-F, Miller TJ. Comparison of Nursing Interventions Classification and Current Procedural Terminology codes for categorizing nursing activities. Image 1997; 29:133-138.

- Holzemer WL, Henry SB, Dawson C, Sousa K, Bain C, Hsieh S-F. An evaluation of the utility of the Home Health Care Classification for categorizing patient problems and nursing interventions from the hospital setting. In: Gerdin U, Tallberg M, Wainwright P (eds.). Nursing Informatics: The Impact of Nursing Knowledge on Health Care Informatics. Stockholm: IOS Press; 1997: 21-26.

- Horsburgh M. Integrating nursing informatics into a basic nursing education programme. In: Hovenga EJS, Hannah KJ, McCormick KA, Ronald JS (eds.). Nursing Informatics '91: Proceedings of the Fourth International Conference on Nursing Use of Computers and Information Science, Melbourne, Australia, April 14-17, 1991. Lecture Notes in Medical Informatics Volume 42: Springer-Verlag, Berlin, Heidelberg: 1991; 634-640.

131

– Hovenga EJS, Hannah KJ, McCormick KA, Ronald JS (eds.). Nursing Informatics '91: Proceedings of the Fourth International Conference on Nursing Use of Computers and Information Science, Melbourne, Australia, April 14-17, 1991. Lecture Notes in Medical Informatics Volume 42: Springer-Verlag, Berlin, Heidelberg; 1991.

– Hoy D, Hardiker N. Representing nursing: The puzzle of language and classification. In: Mortensen RA (ed.). ICNP and Telematic Applications for Nurses in Europe: The Telenurse Experience. IOS Press, Amsterdam; 1999: 66-76.

– Huff SM, Rocha RA, McDonald CJ, et al. Development of the LOINC (Logical Observation Identifier Names and Codes) Vocabulary. J Am Med Inform Assoc 1998: 276-292.

– Humphreys BL, McCray AT, Cheh ML. Evaluating the coverage of controlled health data terminologies: Report on the results of the NLM/AHCPR Large Scale Vocabulary Test. J Am Med Inform Assoc 1997; 4:484-500.

– Humphreys BL, Lindberg DAB, Schoolman HM, Barnett GO. The Unified Medical Language System: An informatics research collaboration. J Am Med Inform Assoc 1998; 5:1-11.

– Ingenerf J. Taxonomic vocabularies in medicine: the intention of usage determines different established structures. In: Greenes RA, Peterson HE, Protti DJ (eds.). Proceedings of MedInfo95. Vancouver, BC: HealthCare Computing & Communications, Canada, Inc; 1995;136-139.

– ISO (International Standards Organization). International Standard ISO 1087: Terminology–Vocabulary. Geneva, Switzerland: International Standards Organization; 1990.

– Kleinbeck SVM. In search of perioperative nursing data elements. AORN J 1996; 63:926-931.

– Lange I, Muñoz M, Aldunce MI, Camus L, Urrutia M (eds.). [The Practice of Nursing in Latin America]. (Article in Spanish). Document Prepared for the W.K.Kellog Foundation International Meeting on the Impact of Nursing in the Health of Latin America and The Caribbean. Belo Horizonte, Brazil; 2000.

– Lange LL. Representation of everyday clinical nursing language in UMLS and SNOMED. In: Cimino JJ (ed.) Proceedings of the AMIA Fall Symposium. Hanley & Belfus Inc., Philadelphia; 1996:140-144.

– Magalini FI, Mencuccini B, Pertoldi F. Use and usability of the ICNP in a MEDIGUARD structured electronic nursing report. In: Mortensen RA (ed.). ICNP and Telematic Applications for Nurses in Europe: The Telenurse Experience. IOS Press Amsterdam; 1999:128-136.

– Mays E, Weida R, Dionne R, et al. Scalable and expressive medical terminologies. In: Cimino JJ (ed.). Proooodings of AMIA 1996 Fall Symposium. Hanley & Belfus Inc., Philadelphia; 1996: 259-63.

– McDaniel AM. Developing and testing a prototype patient care database. Comput Nurs 1997; 15:129-136.

– Mortensen RA, Nielsen GH. Concerted action TELENURSING. In: Henry SB, Holzemer WL, Tallberg M, Grobe SJ (eds.). Informatics: The infrastructure for quality assessment and improvement in nursing. Proceedings of the Fifth International Nursing Informatics Symposium Post-Conference. UC Nursing Press, San Francisco; 1994: 36-45.

– Nielsen GH. Measuring nursing. In: Nursing in Europe. A resource for better health. Geneva: WHO; 1997. (WHO Regional Publications. European Series no. 74): 241-255.

– NCMT (National Convergent Medical Terminology). Concept Modeling Style Guide. Oakland, CA: Kaiser Permanente; 1999.

– O'Neil MJ, Payne C, Read JD. Read Codes Version 3: A user led terminology. Meth Inform Med 1995; 34:187-192.

– Ozbolt JG. From minimum data to maximum impact: Using clinical data to strengthen patient care. Adv Prac Nurs Q 1996; 1(4):62-69.

– Ozbolt JG, Bakken S, Button P, Warren JJ. Toward a reference terminology model for nursing: The 1999 Nursing Vocabulary Summit Conference. In: Saba VK (ed.). Proceedings of NI 2000. Auckland, New Zealand; (in press).

– Parlocha PK, Henry SB. The utility of Georgetown Home Health Classification Systems for coding patient problems and nursing interventions in psychiatric home care. Comput Nurs 1998; 16:45-52.

– Paul SM. Data management in nursing research. In: Hovenga EJS, Hannah KJ, McCormick KA, Ronald JS (eds.). Nursing Informatics '91: Proceedings of the Fourth International Conference on Nursing Use of Computers and Information Science, Melbourne, Australia, April 14-17, 1991. Lecture Notes in Medical Informatics Volume 42: Springer-Verlag, Berlin, Heidelberg: 1991; 562-566.

– Piccolo U, Rienhoff O, Babst T. Implementation of HIS in Germany: social factors affecting the systems training of nurses. In: Hovenga EJS, Hannah KJ, McCormick KA, Ronald JS (eds.). Nursing Informatics '91: Proceedings of the Fourth International Conference on Nursing Use of Computers and Information Science, Melbourne, Australia, April 14-17, 1991. Lecture Notes in Medical Informatics Volume 42: Springer-Verlag, Berlin, Heidelberg: 1991; 197-202.

– Price C, O'Neil M, Bentley TE, Brown PJB. Exploring the ontology of surgical procedures in the Read Thesaurus. Meth Inform Med 1998; 37:420-425.

– Rector AL, Nowlan WA. The GALEN Representation and Integration Language (GRAIL) Kernel, version 1. In: The GALEN Consortium for the EC. Manchester: University of Manchester; 1993.

– Rector AL, Glowinski AJ, Nowlan WA, Rossi-Mori A. Medical concept models and medical records: An approach based on GALEN and PEN & PAD. J Am Med Inform Assoc 1995; 2:19-35.

– Rector AL, Bechhofer S, Goble CA, Horrocks I, Nowlan WA, Solomon WD. The GRAIL concept modeling language for medical terminology. Artif Intel Med 1997; 9:139-171.

– Romano CA, Heller BR. A curriculum model for graduate specialization in nursing informatics. In: Greene RA (ed.). Proceedings of the twelfth Annual Symposium on Computer Applications in Medical Care. Computer Society Press, New York: 1988; 343-349.

– Ronald JS. A collaborative model for specialization in nursing informatics. In: Hovenga EJS, Hannah KJ, McCormick KA, Ronald JS (eds.). Nursing Informatics '91: Proceedings of the Fourth International Conference on Nursing Use of Computers and Information Science, Melbourne, Australia, April 14-17, 1991. Lecture Notes in Medical Informatics Volume 42: Springer-Verlag, Berlin, Heidelberg: 1991; 662-666.

– Rossi Mori A, Consorti F, Galeazzi E. Standards to support development of terminological systems for healthcare telematics. Meth Inform Med 1998; 37:551-563.

– Russler DC, Schadow G, Mead C, Synder T, Quade LM, McDonald CJ. Influences of the Unified Service Action Model on the HL7 Reference Information Model. In: Lorenzi N (ed.). Proceedings of the 1999 AMIA Annual Symposium. Hanley & Belfus Inc., Philadelphia: 1999: 930-934.

– Saba VK. Home health care classification system. In: Hovenga, EJS, Hannah KJ;, McCormick KA, Ronald JS (eds.). Nursing Informatics 91. Proceedings of the Fourth International Conference on Nursing Use of Computers and Information Science. Springer-Verlag, Berlin, Heidelberg: 1991; 397.

– Saba VK. The classification of home health care nursing: Diagnoses and interventions. Caring Magazine 1992; 11(3): 50-56.

– Saba VK, Zuckerman AE. A new home health classification method. Caring Magazine 1992; 11(9): 27-34.

– Slajmer-Japelj M, Filej B, Kersnic P. Slovenian efforts. In: Mortensen RA, ed. ICNP and Telematic Applications for Nurses in Europe: The Telenurse Experience. IOS Press, Amsterdam; 1999: 241-242.

– Sowa J. Conceptual Structures. Addison Wesley: Reading, MA; 1984.

– Spackman KA, Campbell KE, Cote RA. SNOMED RT: A Reference Terminology for health care. In: Masys D (ed.). Proceedings of the 1997 AMIA Annual Fall Symposium. Hanley & Belfus Inc., Philadelphia; 1997: 640-644.

– Spackman KA. Presentation to SNOMED Users Group. Washington, DC; 1999.

– Tackenberg P. Consensus building out of many translations: Coming to an agreement about nursing phenomena and interventions. In: Mortensen RA (ed.). ICNP and Telematic Applications for Nurses in Europe: The Telenurse Experience. IOS Press, Amsterdam; 1999: 185-190.

– Thoroddsen A. Primary health care and ICNP: Data from clinical nursing practice through SAGA. In: Mortensen RA (ed.). ICNP and Telematic Applications for Nurses in Europe: The Telenurse Experience. IOS Press, Amsterdam; 1999: 144-152.

– Tuttle MS, Keck KD, Cole WG, et al. Metaphrase: An aid to the clinical conceptualization and formalization of patient problems in healthcare enterprises. Meth Inform Med 1998; 37:373-83.

– Wagenknecht A, Arnet PA, Borgazzi A, Butel J, Elsig Y, Rougé A, Assimacopoulos A. Tomorrow's nursing: no paperwork? In: Hovenga EJS, Hannah KJ, McCormick KA, Ronald JS (eds.). Nursing Informatics '91: Proceedings of the Fourth International Conference on Nursing Use of Computers and Information Science, Melbourne, Australia, April 14-17, 1991. Lecture Notes in Medical Informatics Volume 42: Springer-Verlag, Berlin, Heidelberg: 1991; 54-59.

– Warren JJ, Mead CN, Button P, Androwich I, Henry SB. Development and evaluation of the Loose Cannon Model of nursing interventions using Unified Modeling Language. In: Lorenzi N (ed.). Proceedings of the 1999 AMIA Annual Symposium. Hanley & Belfus Inc, Philadelphia; 1999:1189.

– Werley HH, Lang NM (eds.). Identification of the Nursing Minimum Data Set. Springer, New York; 1988.

– WHO (World Health Organization). International Statistical Classification of Diseases and Related Health Problems (ICD-10). Geneva, Switzerland; 1992.

– Zingo CA. Strategies and tools for creating a common nursing terminology within a large health maintenance organization. In: Gerdin U, Tallberg M, Wainwright P, (eds.). Proceedings of Nursing Informatics: The Impact of Nursing Knowledge on Health Care Informatics. IOS Press, Stockholm; 1997: 27-31.

APPENDIX 5.

Glossary

Action type: the deed performed by a nursing action as expressed by the verb of action sentences.

Associated category: category standing for a set of associated concepts.

Associated concept: concept connected to a base concept by a link.

Base category: semantic category standing for a homogeneous set of base concepts.

Base concept: concept used systematically as super-ordinate concept in intentional definitions.

Bearer: the diffusion of a nursing phenomenon among entities who or which can be said to have the nursing phenomenon.

Beneficiary: the entity to whose advantage a nursing action is performed.

Body site: anatomical position or location of a nursing phenomenon.

Category: concept chosen to stand for a specified set of subordinate concepts, considered homogeneous.

Classification: vocabulary with the purpose of exhaustive and disjunctive partitioning of objects, e.g., International Classification of Diseases, Nursing Interventions Classification (Saba, 1995a; Saba 1995b; Saba and McCormick, 1996).

Classification scheme: an assignment of objects into groups based upon characteristics that objects have in common, e.g. origin, composition, structure, function, etc. (ISO 11179-1).

Classification system: vocabulary with the purpose of exhaustive and disjunctive partitioning of objects, e.g., International Classification of Diseases, Nursing Interventions Classification.

Closed concept standard: a concept standard where the set of links between categories of concepts is given and where the set of concepts exemplifying categories is fixed.

Closed (proprietary) nursing data standard: a data standard where the recommended set of data is static. Static data sets are composed of closed sets of concepts combined by sets of fixed links according to rules of concept standards. An illustration: nursing data standards issued by ANA are such recommendations of proprietary sets of data depicted by classification systems, for example HHCC, Omaha, NANDA, and NIC.

Concept standard: a standard concerned with rules for the combination of nursing concepts that make up the statements of facts referred to as nursing data. The rules are composed of links connecting categories of concepts. The categories connected by links are exemplified by concepts in the same way as variables connected by functions are exemplified by values.

Concept: unit of thought constituted through abstraction on the basis of properties common to a set of one or more referents. NOTE: This definition is taken from the current revision of ISO CD 1087-1.

Controlled vocabulary: a terminological dictionary containing (and restricted to) the terminology of a specific subject field or of related subject field and based on terminology work. (ISO 1087/CEN ENV 12264).

Data standard: a recommended set of data.

Duration: the length of a time interval during which a nursing phenomenon occurs.

Focus: the area of interest or attention of a nursing phenomenon often expressed in neutral and atomic terms.

Formal terminologies: vocabularies based on concepts (a unit of thought) rather than terms (a unit of language) that include explicit rules for sensible composition of primitive concepts into complex concepts, e.g., SNOMED RT, GALEN.

Frequency: the number of occurrences or repetitions of a nursing phenomenon during a time interval.

Judgment: the clinical opinion, the estimate, or determination regarding the state of nursing phenomena, including the relative quality of the intensity of the manifestation of the nursing phenomenon.

Language: a set of characters, conventions, and rules for conveying information (ANSI X3-172).

Likelihood: the probability of occurrence of a nursing phenomenon.

Link: relation from a base concept.

Location: the anatomical and spatial orientation of an action. Location includes both Body Site defined as anatomical location of a nursing action and Place defined as the spatial location where the nursing action is taking place.

Mean: the entity used in performing a nursing action. Means includes either instruments defined as tools used when performing a nursing action and services defined as specific work or plan used when performing a nursing action.

Nomenclatures: combinatorial vocabularies with the structures organized around polyhierarchies or axes, e.g., SNOMED International, International Classification for Nursing Practice (ICNP). Explicit rules for canonic representations are lacking. It is also defined as a system of designations (terms) elaborated according to pre-established rules (ISO 1087).

Nursing data standard: a standard concerned with the recommendation of sets of data. NOTE: Statements of facts referred to as nursing data are composed of sets of concepts combined by sets of links according to rules of concept standards.

Open concept standard: An open concept standard is a concept standard where the set of links between categories of concepts is variable and where the set of concepts exemplifying categories is unfixed.

Open nursing data standard: a data standard where the recommended set of data is dynamic. Dynamic data sets are composed of open sets of concepts combined by variable sets of links according to rules of concept standards. A dynamic nursing data standard allows users who feel that existing classification systems are lacking in relevance and completeness the opportunity of developing new data standards to be recommended. It is very important to note, that the open approach does not require users of, for example HHCC, NANDA or NIC, to give up their favored nursing classification system because it is simply considered one (static) set of example values in one (static) pre-combined ordering complying with implicit concept standards.

Standards: the National Standards Policy Advisory Committee (USA) defines standards broadly as "a prescribed set of rules, conditions, or requirements concerning definition of terms; classification of components; specification of materials, performance or operations; delineation of procedures; or measurements of quantity and quality in describing materials, products, systems, services or practices" (National Standards Policy Advisory Committee, 1978).

Target (object): the entity that is affected by the nursing action or provides the content of the nursing action.

Taxonomy: a classification according to presumed natural relationships among types and their subtypes (ISO 11179-1).

Term: designation of a defined concept in a special language by a linguistic expression (ISO 1087).

Terminology: the set of terms representing a system of concepts (ISO 1087). According to Ingenerf (1995), Taxonomic Vocabularies can be classified in four types: Thesauri, Classification Systems, Nomenclatures and Formal Terminology

Thesaurus: the vocabulary of a controlled indexing language, formally organized so that a priori relationship between concepts are made explicit; vocabularies based on words, e.g., Medical Subject Heading terms (MeSH) (ISO 2788).

Time: the temporal orientation of a nursing action. Time includes both Time Points (events) defined as definite moments in time and Time Intervals (episodes) defined as the duration between two events.

Topology: the anatomical region in relation to a median point or extent of the anatomical area involved of a nursing phenomenon.

Vocabulary: terms from a subject field and their definition (ISO 1087).